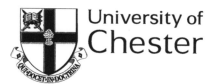

University of
Chester

LIS Library

Chester 01244 511234
Warrington 01925 534284
lis.helpdesk@chester.ac.uk

03

D1437205

CLASS INEQUALITY AND HEALTH CARE

CLASS INEQUALITY AND HEALTH CARE

The Origins and Impact of the National Health Service

VIVIENNE WALTERS

NORTH
CHESHIRE COLLEGE
LIBRARY
ACC. NO. 112,530

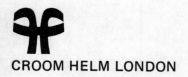

CROOM HELM LONDON

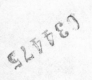

© 1980 Vivienne Walters
Croom Helm Ltd, 2-10 St John's Road, London SW11

ISBN 0-85664-685-7

British Library Cataloguing in Publication Data

Walters, Vivienne
    Class inequality and health care.
    1. Medical care — Great Britain 2. Equality
    3. Great Britain — National Health Service
    I. Title
    362. 1'0941   RA395.G7

    ISBN 0-85664-685-7

Printed and bound in Great Britain by
Redwood Burn Limited
Trowbridge & Esher

CONTENTS

List of Tables

Acknowledgements

Introduction   13

1. The Growth and Impact of Social Welfare Legislation   16

2. Access to Medical Care Before 1948   24

3. Financial and Organisational Problems within the Health Sector   47

4. Working Class Pressures for Reform   61

5. The Medical Profession and Reform of the Health Services   76

6. The Introduction of the NHS   104

7. Class Differences in Needs for Health Care   115

8. Class Differences in Access to General Practitioner Care   129

9. Class Inequality in the Hospital System   142

10. Conclusion   156

Bibliography   163

Index   172

TABLES

6.1: Mean Monthly Sickness, Prevalence and Incapacity Rates by Occupational Groups, Males, England and Wales, 1947

6.2: Mean Monthly Medical Consultation Rates by Sex and Income Group of Chief Wage Earner, 1947 and 1949, and of Head of Household, 1951, England and Wales

7.1: Neo-natal and Post Neo-natal Mortality Rates per 1,000 Legitimate Live Births by Father's Social Class, England and Wales, for Selected Years 1911-50

7.2: Early Neo-natal, Late Neo-natal and Post Neo-natal Mortality Rates per 1,000 Live Births by Sex and Social Class, England and Wales, 1970-2

7.3: Stillbirth Rates per 1,000 Single Births, Standardised for Mother's Age and Parity by Social Class, England and Wales, for Selected Years 1939-72

7.4: Standardised Mortality Ratios for Males by Social Class, England and Wales, for Selected Years 1930-72

7.5: Standardised Mortality Ratios for Death from Four Causes and All Causes for Adult Males Aged 20-64 Years by Social Class, England and Wales 1930-2, 1950 and 1970-2

7.6: Chronic and Acute Illness Rates by Socio-economic Group and Sex, Great Britain, 1974

8.1: Patient Consulting Rates for Children Under 15 Years and Males Aged 15-64 Years by Social Class with Occupational Breakdowns for Classes III, IV and V, May 1955-April 1956

8.2: Mean Monthly Sickness, Prevalence, Incapacity and Medical Consultation Rates per 100 Persons Interviewed by Sex and Weekly Income, England and Wales, 1949 and 1951

8.3: Chronic and Acute Illness and Consultation Rates by Socio-economic Group and Sex, Great Britain, 1975

9.1: Admissions, Mean Duration of Stay and Percentage of Beds Used by Social Class, England and Wales, 1960-1

9.2: Proportionate Distribution by Social Class of Discharges in 1949 from Three Groups of Hospitals Participating in

the General Register Office's Study of Hospital
Morbidity in England and Wales, Males Aged 25-64
Years, All Diagnostic Conditions Excluding Injuries

TO MY PARENTS

ACKNOWLEDGEMENTS

Part of this book is based on my doctoral thesis and I appreciate the criticism and guidance which I received from my adviser, Donald Von Eschen. Critical reactions to early drafts of the book have been valuable and I would like to thank those friends and colleagues who read the manuscript or parts of it: they are Jerry Bull, Barry Edginton, Joe Herbert, Graham Knight and Peta Sheriff. The deficiencies which remain are, of course, my own responsibility. Shirley McGill typed the manuscript and I am grateful for both her patience and her accuracy.

INTRODUCTION

This book is concerned with the introduction and impact of the National Health Service (NHS). In particular, it explores the role which the state has played in reducing class inequalities in health and access to health care. Since its introduction in 1948, the NHS has generally been regarded with veneration and it has been seen as one of the most socialist of the various reforms which comprise the 'welfare state'. By removing most of the direct costs of care, it is assumed that the service has distributed care on the basis of need alone. There is a general belief that, though the service may be deficient in other respects, it has removed class inequalities in access to care and, by implication, reduced inequalities in health.

This image of the NHS coincides with common explanations of the growth and impact of social welfare legislation. Two general arguments have frequently been advanced about the role of the state and the extent to which it alters class relations in contemporary capitalist society. In the first place, it is assumed that social welfare legislation has been enacted in response to the deprivations experienced by the working class and the pressures for reform which arise from these. The state is seen to respond to class conflict by introducing social reforms in an effort to dissipate this conflict and stabilise the society. Second, it is commonly assumed that social welfare legislation achieves some reduction in class inequality. This book questions whether these arguments offer adequate explanations of the introduction and impact of the NHS. Was the service a response to the radicalisation of the working class? Has it reduced class inequalities in health and access to medical care? What I will try to show is that neither of these are appropriate conclusions.

First, we will look at the development of health services in Britain since the mid-nineteenth century and the way in which changes in the organisation of these services affected the access to care of working class and middle class patients. But rather than focusing attention solely on the barriers to care which patients of different social class faced, I will place these in the context of other problems which can also be identified within the health sector. This analysis suggests that the NHS was not so much a response to the difficulties working class patients experienced in obtaining care, as an attempt to rationalise an inefficient

13

health care system and provide it with a stable financial base.

Yet the existence of a broad range of structural and financial problems does not, in itself, lend adequate support to the thesis that the NHS was introduced in order to rationalise the organisation and delivery of health care. We must also look at the deficiencies which were actually being identified within the health sector and at the types of reforms which were seen to be necessary. This leads us into analyses of the ways in which representatives of the working class, the medical profession and the state shaped the debate over reform and defined the need for change. In each case, we are drawn to the conclusion that, rather than being a response to working class demands for reform, the NHS was a response to the increasingly severe organisational and fiscal problems within the health sector. The state was seeking to rationalise the health care system through the creation of a nationally co-ordinated and publicly financed state medical service.

It is difficult to determine whether the NHS distributes care on the basis of need alone. However, using data on class differences in mortality and morbidity as indices of patients' needs for care, I will look at the use which working class and middle class patients have made of two branches of the NHS — general practitioner and hospital services. Also, we will consider variations in the quality of care received by these patients. There are relatively few studies which have explored these issues, for the common assumption that the NHS provides care on the basis of need appears to have inhibited critical research. The available data do not validate this complacency. Yet there is evidence to suggest that the NHS had a minimal effect on the ease with which working class patients obtained health care and that they enjoy less ready access to care than middle class patients. Moreover, class inequalities in mortality rates have not narrowed since the turn of the century; the availability of medical care for working class patients seems to have been ineffective in reducing class inequalities in health.

Such are the specific issues which I will explore in the following chapters. They prompt us, in conclusion, to reconsider the significance of state intervention in the health sector and to question the ways in which health and illness have been defined. These are not simply academic issues, for they have a bearing upon the way in which we approach the problem of illness. Should we continue to see illness as being reduced through appropriate medical intervention and seek to facilitate access to care? If we step beyond this definition, is it sufficient to recognise that illness is linked with the life styles which characterise industrial societies and then attempt to change these by educating people about the value of such things as good nutrition and frequent exercise? Or must we go beyond this and recognise political bases of illness? Consistent class inequalities in mortality and morbidity rates suggest that we should explore the links between illness and social class. It may be that class inequalities in health will only diminish when fundamental changes occur in the structure of class relations in British society.

These issues are seldom debated. Health has generally been equated with the right of all people to have easy access to medical care and the assumption that the NHS provided care on the basis of need alone has led to the mistaken belief that class inequalities in health will diminish. But rather than reducing class inequalities in health and access to care, the state appears to have served an ideological function — by defining health largely as a problem of access to care, it has fostered a belief in the decline of class inequalities.

One final comment is appropriate. I am not assuming that modern medicine is wholly ineffective in coping with the problem of illness. I am simply arguing that it provides us with too narrow a perspective for understanding illness. I am suggesting that in order to explain patterns of illness, we must also examine the links which appear to exist between illness and the structure of class relations in Britain.

1 THE GROWTH AND IMPACT OF SOCIAL WELFARE LEGISLATION

Different themes may be identified in analyses of the growth of social welfare legislation.[1] Some writers, concerned with the impact of 'great men', have argued that the philosophies and doctrines of men of ideas — philosophers, priests, social theorists — have generated change through their influence on public opinion and, ultimately, on law. Here, the realm of ideas is generally seen as having an autonomous existence, relatively untouched by the changing structure of a society experiencing rapid population growth, industrialisation and urbanisation, but capable of changing this structure. Then there are other analyses which bypass the role of ideas in creating social change and focus on the manner in which structural changes in British society created the need for social reforms. The social reforms of the nineteenth century are seen as a response to the inevitable problems produced by industrialisation. Given the fact that problems of widespread poverty, growing social cleavages, mass illiteracy and abominable working conditions threatened the very fabric of society, then state initiated social reforms and the limitation of property rights are seen as social imperatives. In consequence, social welfare legislation is taken to be a functional prerequisite, imperative for the continued existence and development of society.

More recently, writers have emphasised the importance of class interests and the conflicts arising from these in explaining the growth of social welfare legislation. In this work, different lines of argument can be identified. On the one hand, it is argued that social reforms are a palliative introduced by the state, in response to the radicalisation of the working class. As a result, capitalism is stabilised and some gains are made by the working class, though relatively little change occurs in the distribution of class power and privilege.[2] At the same time, social welfare legislation is viewed as a mechanism by which the state ensures the reproduction of labour through maintenance of minimum levels of health, education and income within the working class. Here also, social reforms function to stabilise capitalism and, while the state acts on behalf of the capitalist class or in the interests of capital, the working class does gain certain limited benefits.

On the other hand, departing from Marxist analyses, but retaining an emphasis on class conflict, some sociologists have viewed social reforms as gains wrested from a dominant class. These reforms are then taken to be indicative of the growing power of workers and the emergence of a pluralistic society.[3] Within such a perspective, it is assumed that social welfare legislation is contrary to the interests of the dominant class and results in a redistribution of class power and privilege. The sharp class divisions of capitalism thus give way to a new pluralistic industrial society and, though conflict continues as a result of different interests, the battle is more equal and the future is seen to promise a continuing reduction of inequality. The state is viewed as the mediator between competing interests, often acting against property interests in order to reduce class inequalities.

Despite the fact that it is possible to identify these different themes, social welfare legislation has received relatively little attention from sociologists; general sociological perspectives have been invoked to explain its growth and few of these explanations have been founded on a sound empirical base. As a result, many deductions about the significance of social reforms, the role of the state and the manner in which it alters class relations in contemporary capitalist society, remain at the level of assumptions. In order to lay a framework for the issues discussed in the following chapters, let us look a little more closely at those arguments which have commonly been used to explain the introduction and impact of social reforms, particularly the NHS.

Social Welfare Legislation: A Response to Working Class Pressures for Reform

Overlooking certain differences in detail, we may identify some common themes in analyses of the growth of social welfare legislation. In the first place, many writers have argued that social reforms have been introduced in response to demands from the working class or in anticipation of such demands. For example, Strachey, in his analysis of the 'new stage which capitalism has entered', sees power as no longer being located almost exclusively in the hands of a capitalist class, but as being diffused throughout the community. In his opinion, the state has assumed a more important and more powerful role, responding to and representing the varied interests within British society:

> the House of Commons itself reflects and responds to the diverse, divergent, reciprocating social forces of the whole community. Every section of the British people has found a way of bringing to bear its influence on the making of the government decisions.[4]

For him, the growth of social welfare legislation symbolises the triumph of representative democracy and is an indication of the capacity of the state to act in the interests of wage earners. He views the organisation of workers into trade unions and the competitive bidding of the parties for workers' votes as important reasons for the development of this new stage of capitalism and he comments that, paradoxically, 'it has been . . . the struggle of democratic forces *against* capitalism which has saved the system'.[5]

Miliband's analysis of the state in capitalist society also suggests that social reforms were enacted as a result of pressures from workers. Writing of the NHS and the comprehensive system of social insurance established in Britain in the 1940s, he argues that:

> These measures which were the pillars of the 'Welfare State', represented of course a major, it could even be said a dramatic extension of the system of welfare which was part of the 'ransom' the working classes had been able to extract from their rulers in the course of a hundred years.[6]

Similarly, Wedderburn, in concluding her review of theories of the 'welfare state', implies the importance of the organisation and political action of the working class in determining the growth of social welfare legislation. She writes that, in order to explain differences in the extensiveness of social welfare services and programmes between capitalist societies, we have to look at the political strength of the working class, its success in winning allies from particular pressure and interest groups and its demands for social justice.[7]

This same theme is also central in Navarro's analysis of the NHS. He starts from the position that 'social class is a most necessary category of analysis of social and political behaviour . . . the conflicts and antagonisms among classes are the main determinants . . . of social change.'[8] He argues that 'the nature, functions, composition and distribution of services [within the health sector] and its different components are determined primarily by forces *outside* — not within — it.[9] His thesis is that the NHS was a response to the radicalisation of the working class:

> it is impossible to explain the creation of the NHS in Britain without understanding the relationship of class forces in Britain and the wartime radicalisation of the working class that had called into question 'the survival of capitalism' . . . The much heralded consensus on the need for a national health service that existed among Labour and

Conservative politicians was the result of the radicalisation of the working class on the one hand and the concern for the survival of capitalism by the capitalist class on the other.[10]

Thus, while the NHS was a response to working class pressures and, as such, represented 'a victory for the British working class', Navarro argues that such social reforms also serve the interests of the capitalist class and function to defend the capitalist system by dissipating the social unrest which threatens the survival of the system. A similar thesis is developed by Pivan and Cloward in their study of the welfare 'explosion' of the 1960s in the United States.[11] They conclude that the function of welfare services is to protect the social system by buying off the poor in times of social unrest. By means of example, they chart the growth of the Poor Law system of relief in Britain:

> During the late 18th and early 19th centuries the English countryside was periodically besieged by turbulent masses of the displaced rural poor and the towns were racked by Luddism, radicalism, trade unionism, and Chartism, even while the ruling classes worried about what the French Revolution might augur for England . . . It was at this time that the poor relief system — first created in the 16th century to control the earlier disturbances caused by population growth and the commercialization of agriculture — became a major institution . . . The relief system . . . was expanded in order to absorb and regulate the masses of discontented people uprooted from agriculture but not yet incorporated into industry.[12]

Such observations, drawn from the work of social historians, provide the basis for Pivan and Cloward's analysis of the relief system in the United States. Roosevelt's 'New Deal', for example, is explained not as a response to widespread unemployment, but as a result of the 'rising surge of political unrest that accompanied this economic catastrophe'.[13]

In these ways, the importance of working class demands for reform is emphasised in explanations of the growth of social welfare legislation. What is presupposed in each of these analyses is the advantageous position of the middle class and the deprivation of the working class — deprivation in terms of unemployment, income, health care, schooling and housing. It is around these issues that the working class organises. Moreover, it is implied that welfare measures are addressed, at least partly, to the needs of the working class. Even if reforms are introduced to ensure 'the stabilisation, rationalisation and continued expansion of the existing political economy',[14] they can do so, presumably, only by effecting some change in the conditions of life of the working class. That such a priority was assigned to reducing inequality is implied by Jay when he comments that 'the assault on poverty and inequality through redistribution must *remain* the prime purpose for a very long way ahead'.[15] Similarly, Frankel implies that the social reforms of the 1940s were attempts to prevent the more marked class inequalities and deprivations of the working class in the pre-war years:

> During and after World War II . . . 'Western' governments declared their intention to prevent a return to pre-war evils, and, in this spirit, the British Coalition Government asserted its determination to maintain full employment, to institute comprehensive social services, including secondary education for all, to break down old social barriers and to abolish want and poverty.[16]

But have social reforms actually reduced class inequalities?

Social Welfare Legislation and Class Inequality

Consistent with the assumption that social reforms are directed towards improving the conditions of life of the working class, is the belief that the worst aspects of poverty have been eliminated and inequalities have been reduced by means of taxation, transfer payments and such benefits in kind as free health care and subsidised housing. For over a decade after the Second World War, such beliefs were widespread in Britain. It was not until the 1960s that this optimism gave way to more skeptical questioning and now, we can identify a certain ambivalence towards the achievements of the 'welfare state'. Critical analyses document the continued existence of poverty, the persistence of inequalities in income and wealth and in access to education and health care. Yet such criticism generally goes hand in hand with a recognition, more or less explicit, that without the present welfare services and programmes, class inequalities would be of much greater magnitude. Even if the original hopes of idealists have not been fulfilled, an improvement in the situation of the working class is cautiously recognised.

Some of this ambivalence is captured in Miliband's comments on the 'welfare state' when he writes that it 'did not, for all its importance, constitute any threat to the existing system of power and privilege. What it did constitute was a certain humanisation of the *existing* social order.'[17] While Navarro labels the NHS as a 'very positive victory for the working class', he argues that the implementation of the Act was 'far from the revolutionary advance that it is generally assumed to have been', though it was 'not a minor step in itself'.[18]

An earlier and more positive evaluation may be found in the work of Strachey who notes a reduction in class inequality which, though not marked, is evidence of the strengths of representative democracy, the 'welfare state' and the new power in the hands of workers. He views the future with similar optimism: 'At this point in their development representative institutions are likely to be used by the wage earners to attempt to re-model the economic system in their own interests.'[19] In the early sixties Titmuss argued that the belief that inequalities had been reduced and that 'welfare state' afforded very real protection to the working class against the vicissitudes of life, was widespread.[20] Such beliefs have not been wholly discredited over the past two decades. Thus it is possible for Cochrane to argue that 'it would appear that the NHS has gone a long way towards reducing social class inequality';[21] for Rein to claim that 'lower class patients enjoy easy access to health care';[22] and for Mechanic to conclude that 'one of the most impressive accomplishments of the National Health Service has been to provide care in relation to need rather than in response to the ability to pay'.[23] Of all the social reforms of the 1940s, the NHS has been viewed as the most successful and, not surprisingly, the assumed success of the service has been matched by complacency. Even in critical analyses of British society, the service has been conspicuously ignored. As Rossdale writes, 'more than any other creation of the post-war Labour government, the National Health Service has been regarded with veneration and satisfaction by those on the Left'.[24]

Such optimism is less frequently found in recent analyses of the service. For example, Parker notes class and regional inequalities in health, the provision of health personnel and facilities and the use of health services.[25] She concludes that 'insofar as it is judged in terms of a system which aims to relate medical services to need, the National Health Service must be considered a failure'.[26] Also, Hart elaborates an 'inverse care law', arguing that good medical care is least likely to be available in regions where it is most needed.[27] A healthy scepticism towards the achievements of the NHS is growing, but still, relatively little research is concerned with estimating the success of the service in reducing class inequalities in health and access to care.

Conclusion

Two major assumptions may be identified in analyses of the growth of social welfare legislation. First, it is frequently assumed that state initiated social reforms have been introduced in response to class conflict and in an effort to diffuse this conflict. Second, it is assumed that such reforms achieve a reduction in class inequality. Pluralist analyses of contemporary industrial society tend to be more optimistic in this respect; Marxist analyses more guardedly recognise that benefits flow to the working class as a result of social reforms, for they also argue that no fundamental change occurs in the nature of class relations in capitalist society.

Few writers have challenged the validity of making these assumptions about the introduction and impact of the NHS. Though criticisms have been made of the organisation of health services and of the quality of care provided for patients, it has generally been assumed that care is now distributed on the basis of need alone. Coupled with this assumption is the belief that, prior to the introduction of the service, working class patients were disadvantaged in their access to care whereas middle class patients enjoyed comparatively easy access to care. The following chapters question these assumptions.[28] Was the NHS a response to the poor access to care of working class patients? Was the organised working class pressing for reform of the health services? Has the NHS achieved a reduction in class inequalities in health and access to care? In other words, to what extent is the NHS an indication of the state's role in diffusing class conflict by acceding to the demands of the working class and narrowing class inequalities?

Notes

1. For a discussion of explanations of the growth of social welfare legislation see John H. Goldthorpe, 'The Development of Social Policy in England, 1800-1914', *Transactions of the Fifth World Congress of Sociology*, vol. IV (1964).

2 Vicente Navarro, *Class Struggle, The State and Medicine* (Martin Robertson, London, 1978); Navarro, 'Social Class, Political Power and the State and Their Implications in Medicine', *Social Science and Medicine*, vol. 10 (1976), pp. 437-57; N. Birnbaum, *The Crisis of Industrial Society* (Oxford University Press, London, 1969); R. Miliband, *The State in Capitalist Society* (Quartet, London, 1969); J. Weinstein, *The Corporate Ideal in the Liberal State* (Beacon Press, Boston, 1968).

3. A. Rose, *The Power Structure* (Oxford University Press, New York, 1967); D. Jay, *Socialism in the New Society* (Longmans, London, 1962); J. Strachey, *Contemporary Capitalism* (Victor Gollancz, London, 1956).

4. Strachey, *Contemporary Capitalism*, p. 73.

5. Ibid., p. 154.

6. Miliband, *The State in Capitalist Society*, p. 99.

7. Dorothy Wedderburn, 'Facts and Theories of the Welfare State', *The Socialist Register* (1965), pp. 142-3.

8. Navarro, *Class Struggle, The State and Medicine*, p. xiv.

9. Ibid.

10. Navarro, 'Social Class, Political Power and the State and Their Implications in Medicine', p. 452.

11. Frances Fox Pivan and Richard A. Cloward, *Regulating the Poor: The Functions of Public Welfare* (Pantheon Books, New York, 1971).

12. Ibid., pp. 20-1.

13. Ibid., p. 45.

14. Weinstein, *The Corporate Ideal in the Liberal State*, p. ix.

15. Jay, *Socialism in the New Society*, p. 224 (emphasis mine).

16. H. Frankel, *Capitalist Society and Modern Sociology* (Lawrence and Wishart, London, 1970), p. 69.

17. Miliband, *The State in Capitalist Society*, p. 99.

18. Navarro, *Class Struggle, The State and Medicine*, p. 47.

19. Strachey, *Contemporary Capitalism*, p. 160.

20. Richard M. Titmuss, *Essays on the Welfare State*(Unwin University Books, London, 1963), pp. 34-9.

21. A.L. Cochrane, *Effectiveness and Efficiency* (Nuffield Provincial Hospitals Trust, London, 1972), p. 71.

22. M. Rein, 'Social Class and the Utilization of Medical Care Services', *Hospitals*, vol. 43 (1 July 1969), pp. 43-54.

23. D. Mechanic, 'The English National Health Service: Some Comparisons With the United States', *Journal of Health and Social Behaviour*, vol. 12 (1971), pp. 22-3.

24. M. Rossdale, 'Socialist Health Service?' *New Left Review*, no. 36 (1966), p. 3.

25. Julia Parker, *Social Policy and Citizenship* (Macmillan, London, 1975).

26. Ibid., p. 82.

27. Julian Tudor Hart, 'The Inverse Care Law', *Lancet*, i (1971), pp. 405-12.

28. I define classes in terms of their relationship to the production process. The working class is comprised of wage-earners employed in manual labour and the middle class is made up of largely salaried non-manual workers and their families. Dominating these classes is an upper class composed of the land owning aristocracy and the owners of financial and industrial capital. For an analysis of the class structure of British society, see John Westergaard and Henrietta Resler, *Class in a Capitalist Society* (Penguin, Harmondsworth, 1976).

2   ACCESS TO MEDICAL CARE BEFORE 1948

Even a cursory glance at the organisation of health services before 1948 suggests that it is wrong to assume that working class patients were singularly disadvantaged in their access to health care. If we first turn our attention back to the mid-nineteenth century we see that the source from which patients obtained medical care was largely determined by their class position. Care was provided at all levels of the class hierarchy and, in theory at least, a patient's ability to pay did not determine whether or not a doctor was consulted when the need arose; it simply dictated the organisational context in which he or she would receive treatment. Accounts of the types of care provided by the different sources suggest wide differences in quality and indicate that working class patients, particularly the destitute, obtained care of distinctly lesser quality than middle class, fee paying patients. Also, it is possible that working class patients made much less use of the services which were available to them. But such class inequalities in the use of services and quality of care at that point in time did not really matter, since medicine had little impact on the quality of health which people experienced and it was not, as yet, a highly valued commodity. Class differences in access to care were not an important aspect of class inequality and little sense of deprivation arose from these differences.

Sources of Medical Care in the Mid-Nineteenth Century

A patient's ability to pay for care determined the source from which it was obtained.[1] Middle and high income families received care in their homes as private fee paying patients — even surgical procedures would be performed at home, perhaps on a well scrubbed kitchen table. Given the poor conditions existing in the hospitals of the time, this was infintely preferable to institutional care. The wealthy were attended by the elite of the medical profession — fellows and licentiates of the Royal College of Physicians and licentiates of the College of Surgeons — and the less affluent were treated by general practitioners. Physicians' fees were generally graded in accordance with a patient's income or yearly house rental and in this manner a process of income redistribution operated. Patients with an annual income over £500 were charged one guinea for a single visit while those with incomes under £100 were charged only 2s.6d. For patients with an annual rental over £100, attendance at childbirth cost five guineas or more, whereas those paying a rent of £10-25 were charged one guinea.[2] Wealthy patients thus subsidised the care of lower income families and physicians were able to offer their services to working class patients at little or no cost.

While more affluent patients were attended in their homes, low income and destitute patients obtained care in a variety of different settings. Hospital care was provided mainly for the working class, most especially for the destitute. In the mid-nineteenth century, medical science was still in its infancy and hospitals had little effect on mortality rates except by isolating and eventually eradicating more virulent diseases. Even Florence Nightingale's first requirement — that hospitals should at least do no harm to patients — was only infrequently met and patients operated on at home were more likely to recover and to recover sooner than if they had been hospitalised.[3] It is understandable, therefore, that hospitals were essentially working class institutions, particularly since middle class patients could afford to pay for private treatment at home and for nursing and domestic help.

Free care was provided by the voluntary hospitals and through the Poor Law. The former dealt largely with acute cases while the latter catered to the chronic sick. Indoor medical relief under the Poor Law meant the workhouse, and though the care varied, it was generally poor. There was no separation of patients on the basis of symptoms; the acute sick, the pregnant, the insane, the tuberculous, and mentally defective were all housed together, often in one room. The workhouses were crowded; beds were shared (together with bed bugs); towels were shared; the food was poor and inadequate; sometimes inmates would act as nurses, and the doctors were hired by competition for the lowest price. Coe describes the appalling conditions in these hospitals at this time as follows:

Not only were hospitals typically dirty and poorly ventilated but they were often extremely over-crowded. Each ward was usually filled to capacity with beds lined side by side with barely sufficient space to pass between them. Frequently, more than one patient was placed in a single bed, usually without regard to type of disease or condition of the patient. All too often one's bed partner might have died and the body remained for several hours before being removed by the staff. Thus patients with infectious diseases, patients with gangrenous limbs and those crazed with fever all could be in the same ward . . . all treatments were carried out in the ward including surgery (limited mostly to amputations), physical restraint of the

mentally ill, delivery of an infant, and laying out of the dead. To add
to the patients' miseries the attending physicians and surgeons gener-
aly ignored even the most rudimentary rules of sanitation . . . [4]

Conditions in voluntary hospitals were somewhat better but still, those
who could, shunned the hospitals — to be admitted was almost akin to
a death warrant.

Ambulatory care for working class families was available from
several different sources. Workers often provided for themselves
through membership in a variety of schemes in which treatment from
general practitioners could be wholly or partially paid for by means of
regular weekly contributions. Medical clubs, provident dispensaries, and
provident medical associations all provided care to members who paid
contributions on a regular basis. These were organised by friendly
societies, trade unions, groups of doctors, or employers who contracted
doctors for their employees. Membership in the schemes was not
expensive — contributions to medical clubs ranged from 1d. to 1½d.
per person, while family clubs provided coverage for the whole family
(excluding mid-wifery) for 3d. a week. Friendly societies were among
the most important working class organisations, with more members
than either trade unions or co-operative societies.[5] They charged
workers between 2s.6d. and 3s.0d. a year and provided sickness payments, medical attendance and, in many cases, medicine. It is estimated
that in 1872, they had a total membership of approximately four
million,[6] and by 1905, six million, with funds totalling £40 million.[7]
But even with a considerable growth in such schemes, less than half of
the working population were even moderately covered against the
impact of illness. In fact, there existed several barriers to membership
in these various schemes. Many friendly societies did not cover women
and children, and most schemes did not admit 'bad lives' or those
suffering from constitutional defects or chronic disease. In many
medical clubs, there was no obligation to continue the membership of
those who developed chronic disease, and if the level of illness became
too high, the doctor might discontinue the scheme. Thus, those most
in need of care were often excluded, and if unable to pay the fees
charged a private patient, they were forced to rely on charity and the
Poor Law.

It was the Poor Law which provided non-institutional care for those
at the base of the class hierarchy — the destitute. Treatment was available from District Medical Officers appointed by the Board of
Guardians within each Poor Law Union, but while care was provided

by the District Medical Officer, the pivot of the whole organisation was the Relieving Officer. He, with no medical qualifications, was the executive authority and was responsible for issuing the medical orders without which no one could obtain care. Many deterrents were built into this system; the Relieving Officer was not always easily accessible — in a rural Union, it might be a journey of six or eight miles to reach him — and those applying for medical orders were frequently treated as paupers rather than as patients.[8] Only the destitute were eligible for care and thus, 'in some Unions the applicant for a Medical Order . . . [was] required to attend personally before the Guardians at their meeting, and explain, at the cost of half a day's earnings, how he . . . [came] to need medical aid'.[9] Yet despite such barriers to obtaining treatment, Hodgkinson has argued that unqualified condemnation of the Poor Law is unjust since 'in great sections of the country the Poor Law provided medical aid far superior to what the poor could procure for themselves'.[10] The Webbs also claimed that criticisms of the system of outdoor medical relief failed to do justice to the kindness and hard work of the District Medical Officers.[11]

The deterrents to obtaining care under the Poor Law were mitigated to some extent, by the treatment available at the out-patient departments of the voluntary hospitals. Here, there was almost unrestricted access to care. The whole ethos of the voluntary hospitals was quite different from that underlying the Poor Law. While the latter provided care only to the destitute in order to encourage self-help among the poor, the former were the representatives of a tradition of charitable provision of care for those in need, with no means tests involved. For this reason, they catered to families above and below the level of destitution. But the care was hardly superior to that obtained under the Poor Law; waiting rooms were crowded and treatment hurried, with no time for doctors to consider the patient's problems in detail, unless the case was unusual and particularly interesting for teaching purposes. For the majority of patients, there was a long wait for a repeat of the same old bottle of medicine irrespective of its medical benefits. The psychological effect of such may have been beneficial, yet to conclude that there were any real preventive or curative effects would be a delusion.

There were other sources which provided charitable care for workers and their families, yet these shared many of the same disadvantages. For example, free dispensaries and medical missions abounded in the slum districts of large towns, but the care which was provided was often poor. Only superficial attention was given to patients and the doctors were unable to offer immediate institutional treatment to those in need of it. At its most extreme, philanthropy motivated such inappropriate and indiscriminate care as that of the carriage borne lady who sought to relieve the lot of the poor in one area by 'promiscuously' distributing a dozen half bottles of champagne and a dozen bunches of grapes![12]

The source from which people obtained medical treatment was, therefore, dependent on their class. Clearly, working class patients were not denied care. While middle class patients received private care in their own homes, working class families could obtain medical attention from several other sources; general practitioners charged lower fees for their less affluent patients, the Poor Law provided both indoor and outdoor relief and workers themselves provided for their own treatment through a variety of schemes organised by friendly societies, trade unions, doctors, employers and philanthropists. Unfortunately there are no data on the actual rates of use of these services by patients of different social class. Indeed, working class patients may have made much less use of the services than their needs for care warranted. The Webbs noted that 'In the slums of the great towns there appear to be many of the poorest families who are completely unaware of their right to obtain free medical attendance, or unacquainted with the formalities necessary to procure it.'[13] And 'in some parts of the country a very large proportion of the cases of sickness . . . [went] without any medical treatment whatsoever'.[14] Moreover, the conditions under which working class and destitute patients received treatment were often quite horrifying. Understandably, people lived in fear of ending up in the workhouse, for the sick poor were by no means exempt from its harsh and repressive life — fears of malingering were always uppermost in the minds of the staff. In order to discourage all but those who were absolutely unable to obtain work and maintain themselves, the life of the workhouse was designed to be infinitely less attractive than the lot of the least fortunate souls who remained outside.

But despite reports of families which received no medical attention and despite accounts of the abysmal conditions under which others obtained treatment, it is doubtful whether inequalities in access to care and in the quality of care were of much significance for people's health. They may have affected the dignity with which people could live their lives and in turn die, but in terms of improving the health of patients, medical care was of as little significance for the destitute as for the wealthy patient. Medicine had relatively little to offer people even in the late nineteenth century. The 1880s marked a turning point in the understanding and treatment of disease, but it was many years before these discoveries were incorporated into the day-to-day care and treatment offered by doctors and hospitals.[15] The efficacy of the actual medical treatment obtained from different sources was unlikely to vary widely. Even though the rich received care from the elite of the medical profession, the treatment was not likely to be very sophisticated. Fellows and licentiates of the Royal College of Surgeons were not always highly qualified practitioners:

> As late as 1834, membership of the College could be obtained for a down payment of fifty guineas after three examinations lasting some twenty minutes each. A man could pass the examination 'who is a good classical scholar but knows nothing of chemistry, little or nothing of anatomy, nothing of the diseases of women in childbed, and nothing of the manner of delivering them'.[16]

Fee-paying patients may have had more time with their doctors and the benefit of talking to a sympathetic listener, but otherwise, the treatment they received was unlikely to be much superior to the popular bottle of medicine dispensed by medical officers, free dispensaries, and voluntary hospitals alike.

Thus it was that differences in the availability and quality of care were of little significance for people's health. Medical science was still in its infancy, and compared to the 1970s, treatment uniformly lacked sophistication. Insofar as medicine had relatively little to offer patients in the mid-nineteenth century, and inasmuch as people endured illness with a sense of fatalism, inequality in access to care was not an important dimension of class inequality at this time. It became more important when medical care became a valued commodity — when people's attitudes towards health grew less passive, and when treatment increased in sophistication.[17] In other words, people's health depended little on whether they received treatment, and they may have felt no sense of deprivation if they could not or did not consult a doctor. However, views of health and illness started to change during the latter part of the nineteenth century and these changes were paralleled and reinforced by major developments in medical science and rapid innovation in the field of medical technology. This was of consequence for both middle class and working class patients and as a result of these changes, inequality of access to health care became a more important dimension of class inequality.

Developments in Medical Science and Changing Perceptions of Health

The rise of the industrial bourgeoisie and their growing prosperity produced a prosperous and expanding clientele for the medical profession.
But the increasing demand for medical care on the part of the middle
and upper classes did not only depend on the fact that they had more
money to spend, it also stemmed from their altered perception of health
and medicine.[18] As the ability to control nature increased, so also the
middle class saw their own bodies as being more subject to control. The
fatalism with which illness had been borne started to decline; less frequently was disease viewed as a punishment for sin or just an unavoid-
able aspect of life. The belief in progress, seemingly confirmed by increasing productivity, produced gradual changes in the attitudes toward
health among the Victorian middle class. Coupled with the idea of progress was the notion of individualism and the emphasis on success and
self-help also served to generate new attitudes toward health and an
increase in the demand for medical care; the more we think is expected
of us in fulfilling our various roles, the more concerned we are likely to
be with the quality of our health. Illness can prevent such fulfilment.
Samuel Smiles, the 'apostle of self-help', writing in the mid-nineteenth
century was emphatic about the close connection between good health
and the attainment of wordly success.[19] 'Practical success in life', he
noted, 'depends more upon physical health than is generally
imagined'.[20] He showed how successful men had also been very
healthy, and argued that the 'success of even professional men depends
in no slight degree upon their physical health'.[21] In these ways attitudes
towards health were linked with the ideology of industrial capitalism
and people were taught the importance of good health in increasing
their chances of success.

  This transition in perceptions of health and illness was in no small
part due to the changes which were occurring in medical science and to
the achievements claimed by the medical profession. The profession
had for centuries been slowly freeing itself from the religious
dogmatism of medieval times, but it was not until the last decades of
the nineteenth century that major discoveries were made and rapid
changes took place in the diagnosis and treatment of disease. It was
some time before these were assimilated into the actual practice of
medicine, but the new promise which the profession offered, a promise
of more effective, scientific medicine, helped to further stimulate the
demand for medical care. The elite of the profession encouraged the
continued growth of specialisation and this, together with the developing medical technology, vastly increased the costs of providing care.

As a consequence of these changes, the hospitals provided more and more sophisticated care and assumed an increasingly important role within the total health system, and since this care also became more costly, charges for hospital care were introduced. Because middle class and working class patients received care from different sources, the significance of these changes was different for each class.

Working Class Patients: An Increased Demand for Hospital Care

The reorganisation of the Poor Law in 1834 had provided for a national approach by allowing for central direction of policy and by the early twentieth century, the national government had assumed a greater role in the provision of health care. The way was paved for change by the Metropolitan Poor Act of 1867 and the Poor Law Amendment Act of 1868. These Acts empowered London and the provincial unions to provide separate infirmaries for their destitute sick, and they were the first explicit acknowledgement that it was the duty of the government to provide hospitals for the poor. As such, they represent an important step toward the creation of the NHS. Not all unions built separate infirmaries, but where these were established, they were generally far superior to the workhouse facilities in terms of design, staff, and equipment. Indeed some people voiced their apprehension that the high quality of care and expensive treatment might act as an incentive for people to become paupers in order to qualify for treatment.[22]

With the establishment of separate infirmaries, the stigma attached to accepting hospital care under the Poor Law slowly disappeared and people started to make a distinction between the workhouse and the infirmary.[23] As a result of the higher quality of care and improvements in conditions, patients above the level of destitution were seeking hospital treatment more frequently and by the 1890s the Poor Law infirmaries were admitting some patients of the non-pauper class. The Poor Law was treating under the common designation of pauper, a range of people

> varying from those miserables whom nothing but the imminent approach of starvation drives into the hated general mixed work-house up to the domestic servants of the wealthy, the highest grades of skilled artisans and even the lower middle class who now claim as a right the attractive ministrations of the rate-maintained Poor Law hospitals characteristic of some of the great towns.[24]

In those cases where patients were not paupers, attempts were made (not always successfully) to regain at least part of the costs of care.

The Metropolitan Poor Act of 1867 assigned the responsibility for providing London with hospitals for indigent fever and smallpox cases to the Metropolitan Asylums Board and though care was supposed to be provided for the pauper class alone, the demand for care was not so limited. In the smallpox epidemic of 1871-2, over one-third of the patients in these hospitals were not paupers at the time of admission. In 1871, 82 per cent of the patients in the Hampstead Hospital were in gainful employment, the majority as skilled artisans. And a similar situation prevailed in the epidemic of 1876-7; about 90 per cent of patients in the Metropolitan Asylums Board hospitals had never received poor relief before.[25]

The Poor Law hospitals provided the bulk of care — in many areas the workhouse or infirmary was the only source of care. In larger towns, there was usually a choice between a Poor Law infirmary and a voluntary hospital, but the former generally provided the majority of beds. In 1906 in London, for example, there were 16,300 infirmary beds and 10,224 in voluntary hospitals. In Liverpool, the number of beds was 2,000 and 1,172 respectively and in Birmingham, 2,200 and 838.[26] The voluntary hospitals were more likely to deal with acute, unique, and medically interesting cases while chronic cases were cared for under the Poor Law. While they provided care for many people of the same status as were treated under the Poor Law, they were also admitting more patients of higher social class and more frequently served patients above the level of destitution. A census of inpatients at the London Hospital on 28 November 1906 revealed that 60 per cent of the hospital population were neither paupers nor on the verge of pauperism.[27]

The Introduction of Charges for Hospital Treatment

In the light of rising costs of care and the growing number of patients above the level of destitution, hospitals started to introduce charges for treatment. Toward the turn of the century, there was a growing concern expressed at the amount of free care available to patients when a portion of these could afford to pay at least something toward the cost of their treatment and by 1890, many London hospitals were taking steps to reduce the number of outpatients who were being treated free of charge. Efforts were less strenuous in the provinces, but here also, attempts were made to limit cases and exclude those who could afford to pay for care. The voluntary hospitals were caught in a dilemma; they needed to minimise demands on their resources, but they also needed large numbers of outpatients as this would help in their appeals for funds, and would also provide a large pool from which to select interesting cases. They could have extended the system of charges which some hospitals operated, but this would have invited protests from general practitioners. Yet the easy dispensation of free care also invited protests. The doctors feared the competition which the hospitals could provide, it was in their interests that the hospitals provided free care, but only to those unable to pay a doctor. So in the 1890s, hospital almoners were employed in checking whether patients could afford to pay toward the cost of their treatment. It is noted in the Royal Commission of 1909 that the almoner of Westminster Hospital in London estimated that in 1903, 1904, and 1905, approximately 15.6 per cent, 13.6 per cent and 17.2 per cent of patients might have arranged for their own treatment through a provident dispensary, friendly society or such like.[28]

It was the Poor Law infirmaries (or, as they later became, the local authority hospitals) which were the most likely to screen patients and submit them to some form of means test.[29] Unlike the voluntary hospitals, they were not in need of interesting cases for teaching purposes, and they had separate services under the Poor Law for those who could not afford the fees of a doctor. But by the end of 1920, most London hospitals had adopted a system of payment by the patients or were considering doing so. Their strained finances, and the move to patients paying at least part of the costs of care was reflected in the change in the role of almoners. Whereas they had previously checked patients whom they thought might be able to pay for care, now they were checking those who claimed they could not.[30] The voluntary hospitals, which had been largely charitable institutions serving the sick poor, were now becoming primarily business concerns. The increase in paying patients is reflected in the proportion of the current income of London teaching hospitals which such payments represented. In 1920, payments by patients accounted for 10 per cent of their current income, and in 1921, 25 per cent.[31] In the 1930s there was a continuing increase in the numbers of patients paying the full costs of care and in funds from pre-insurance schemes; by the eve of the Second World War, approximately 50 per cent of the costs of the voluntary hospitals was paid for by patients.[32]

The Growth of Contributory Schemes

This decline in the availability of free charitable and public care prompted a growth in contributory schemes. There was a marked growth in such schemes after 1870 when deterrents to obtaining relief under the Poor Law were increased, and the voluntary hospitals were starting to restrict the number of patients treated free of charge. As the hospitals' needs for funds grew, their efforts to charge people for at least a part of the cost of their treatment were strengthened and during the 1920s and 1930s, in response to the growing financial problems of the hospitals, there was again a rapid growth in the contributory schemes designed to provide hospital care for workers above the level of destitution.

The largest of these schemes was the Hospital Savings Association which in 1924 had 62,000 contributors and which had grown to 650,000 only five years later.[33] In this, members made a weekly contribution of 3d and were guaranteed general hospital care for no further payment. Most schemes had income limits, but the efforts of the British Medical Association (BMA) to establish such (since they would otherwise be a threat to private practice) were not always successful. A BMA enquiry in 1930 showed that of the contributory plans in operation in 352 hospitals, 237 operated an income limit.[34] The members of these schemes were, in the main, drawn from those sections of the working class with regular jobs, wages above the minimum, and families of modest size.[35] Apart from spreading the costs of obtaining medical care, the main reason for joining contributory plans appears to have been the desire to avoid means tests when seeking treatment. The Political and Economic Planning report on the British Health services in the 1930s indicated that:

> the working classes are prepared to pay considerable premiums for medical insurance without any forms of means test. Insurance payments are popular, but means tests, however mild, have become odious. Hence the extraordinary popularity of hospitals contributory schemes, with nearly five and a quarter million subscribers of between twopence and fourpence a week.[36]

Thus, we see that though free hospital care was less easy to obtain, working class patients continued to have access to relatively low cost medical care during the early decades of the twentieth century. Hospitals opened their doors to a wider spectrum of the working class, and though limitations were increasingly placed on the availability of free care, these were in part counter-balanced by the growth in contributory schemes providing hospital and general medical care. These contributory plans drew their membership largely from the working class.

Middle Class Patients: A Frustrated Demand for Hospital Care

During the mid-nineteenth century middle class patients showed little inclination to enter hospitals and by paying inflated consulation fees, they subsidised the care of those patients using the voluntary hospitals. Towards the turn of the century though, the greatly improved quality of hospital care prompted a greater willingness of patients to be hospitalised and there was a growing recognition of the new demand for care from the middle class. This, coupled with the fact that the voluntary hospitals were facing financial problems, meant that there was an incentive to start admitting paying patients. In 1881, St Thomas's Hospital started to treat paying patients and in 1884, Guy's Hospital followed its lead. By 1890, five of the eleven London teaching hospitals were admitting paying patients and their payments accounted for 5 per cent of the income of the London hospitals.[37]

Such provision of pay beds was relatively small and yet the demand for hospital care continued to increase, particularly after the First World War when fewer families could afford domestic help to care for the sick at home. In an address on 'The Present Position of the Voluntary Hospitals' in 1927, a consultant at St Mary's Hospital noted that 'A class is clamouring for treatment in voluntary hospitals which was never willing previously to consider such treatment as a possibility, and the necessity to meet the demands of the middle class for hospital services has become very insistent.'[38] He emphasised the fact that compared with others, the middle class were particularly disadvantaged in their access to good quality medical care:

It has always been something of an anomaly that the best medical attention in this country under present conditions can be obtained only by two classes, the rich and the poor, and both classes are attended to by practically the same medical advisors . . . But the middle class remains outside this system altogether. The conditions of modern medicine, which necessarily entail team work — that is to say, the examination of the patient by numerous specialists — deprive the middle class patient, as a rule of the full benefits of proper examination and consequently of proper treatment.[39]

Despite the fact that hospitals had opened wards for paying patients, there was general agreement that these barely met the needs of middle class patients. In an address on 'The Voluntary Hospital and Its Future' in 1927, Hogarth, the President of the BMA commented, ' . . . but fancy, five paying beds for the whole of Liverpool! At Brighton there are 14 private rooms, at Colchester 12, and so on. The scale is utterly and grotesquely inadequate.'[40] And *Lancet*, reporting on the enquiry of the King Edward's Hospital Fund into the provision of pay beds in the London area, noted that:

> There is no uniformity about the fees paid nor do the charges always cover the same services nor are the arrangements speaking generally comparable; but it is perfectly clear that the demand of the public for these beds under one set of conditions or another is quite unsatisfied and many witnesses testified to the Committee that a far larger provision of pay beds is necessary as a valuable adjunct to all forms of practice.[41]

The number of pay beds increased throughout the 1920s. In the area covered by the King Edward's Fund it rose from a total of 590 beds in 1920 to 1,055 in 1927.[42] But the scale of provision was still considered to be inadequate and the disadvantaged situation of middle class patients continued to be an issue during the thirties. In a discussion on the future of nursing homes and private wards in hospitals one physician noted that the small number of pay beds 'hardly touch the problem of the patient of moderate means' and was of the opinion that 'The problem of accommodation for middle class patients was . . . likely to increase rather than diminish.'[43] Another argued that 'a great deal was done for the working classes but little for the professional and middle classes'.[44] The King Edward's Fund pledged itself to further increase the number of beds for middle class patients by finding a way to 'give all hospitals the powers now possessed by many of them of providing paying beds for those who could not otherwise obtain treatment'.[45] One physician felt that about three times as many beds were needed as were provided,[46] but by 1935 there were only 1,997 pay beds in the London area.[47] The number of beds would increase in the future: in 1934, for example, Guy's Hospital, which had opened its first ward for paying patients fifty years earlier, laid the foundation stone for a new block for 73 pay beds;[48] the Manchester Royal Infirmary had collected £95,000 over the past two years and was about to start construction of a block for paying patients;[49] J.D. Player donated £25,000 for a block of pay beds at Nottingham General Hospital and Lord Woolavington gave £10,000 towards the cost of establishing pay beds for patients of 'moderate means' at the London

Hospital.[50] But despite a continuing increase in the number of pay beds, middle class patients continued to experience problems in access to hospital care.[51] Not until the introduction of the NHS were these barriers removed.

The problems of middle class patients stemmed in part from the low provision of pay beds in the major hospitals, but they were compounded by the increasing expense of hospital care:

> For the average middle class man a major operation for an acute illness is a financial disaster from which it may take him years to recover. Nowadays it is expensive to be born and often not less expensive to die, but a prolonged recovery is more costly still. These conditions have come about from the change in medical practice; it is no longer possible for one man to deal faithfully with any but the simplest medical cases and the provision of many experts is necessarily expensive.[52]

The enquiry of the King Edward's Fund into the provision of pay beds indicated that 'with the development of expensive methods of treatment and diagnosis a large number of the middle and professional classes are now unable to pay the full cost of services, some of which are often difficult to obtain outside hospitals'.[53] To help people cope with such financial problems, hospitals inaugerated subscription schemes which would spread the costs of care. Most schemes imposed income limits and catered mainly to the working class. For example, the Hospital Savings Association was confined to people with incomes not exceeding £4 for a single person, £5 for a married couple and £6 for a couple with children under sixteen. Yet this was not true of all schemes. The British Provident Association had pioneered a prepayment plan for persons whose incomes exceeded these limits and, despite the opposition of physicians, individual hospitals and groups of hospitals sponsored similar plans. In 1932, for example, King's College Hospital introduced a scheme with no income limits in which patients received 21 days free treatment in a private ward at the hospital. A single person paid one guinea, a married couple, one and a half guineas and a couple with children under 16 years of age, two guineas.[54] Liverpool introduced a scheme in 1934 which covered the costs of a private bed and treatment in a hospital or a co-operating nursing home for 21 days. For single members with an annual income under £400, for members with an income less than £500 a year and with one dependent, and for those with two or more dependents who were earning less

than £600 a year, the cost was one shilling a week.[55] The scheme anticipated a membership of at least 10,000. But the growth of such plans
was slow, partly because of opposition from consultants who saw them
as threatening private consulting practice outside the hospitals.

Only a few physicians denied the increasing problems of middle class
patients in securing adequate health care. One of their number 'thought
that the demand for middle class hospital provision had been exagger-
ated, although he was prepared to admit that it existed. The disadvantages of such a service included the red tape, the lack of the personal
touch and the loss of contact with the family practitioner which institutional treatment involved'.[56] But most physicians were not of this
opinion and the profession sought to devise possible remedies for the
problem. In 1927 the President of the BMA spoke thus:

> I invite you to conceive of your own general hospital here in
> Nottingham, as the hospital of the whole community in the wide
> area which it serves. Conceive it as the hospital not of the poor
> alone, nor yet of the poor and the wide range of middle classes, but
> of all classes who are sick — all who care to use it, with no distinc-
> tion of rich and poor . . . I am not proposing to rob the poor of the
> least part of the birthright bequeathed to them by a long line of
> magnanimous benefactors . . . For the poor the healing given by the
> hospital must still be without money and without price. But why, if
> nothing but the best is good enough for the poor should less than the
> best be offered to others?[57]

But the BMA favoured the admission of private patients to voluntary hospitals only if their physicians could continue to treat them or
supervise their care. Yet hospitals and consultants were unwilling to
extend such privileges to general practitioners because, they argued, it
would lower the standards of care. Furthermore, even though fee
paying patients helped to ease the immediate financial problems of the
hospitals, they were reluctant to admit patients on an extensive scale
for fear that this might jeopardise their efforts to preserve an image as
charitable institutions. They were fearful of anything which might deter
charitable contributions. In addition, some hospitals were prevented
from introducing pay beds by restrictions imposed by charitable trusts.
Many hospitals managed to circumvent these problems, but while the
provision of pay beds increased during the 1930s it was still considered
to be inadequate, and in order to meet the growing demand for hospital
care from the middle class, separate nursing homes and home hospitals

sprang up near the major hospitals.

The medical profession generally favoured this manner of providing institutional care for the middle class. In 1927, *Lancet* commented:

> We have often set out the difficulties which have to be overcome when a charitable foundation created to serve the sick poor accepts patients from another class; these difficulties do not arise when hospitals are designed exclusively . . . for the treatment of the professional and middle classes.[58]

In 1891, there were approximately 9,500 beds in nursing and convalescent homes in England and Wales and by 1911, the total had risen to about 13,000 and by 1921, to 40,000.[59] The provision of private beds was higher in nursing homes than in the voluntary and public hospitals combined. Toward the end of the 1920s it was estimated that there were 3,000 to 4,000 nursing home beds in the London area compared to about 1,000 private beds in voluntary hospitals.[60]

But conditions in these private nursing homes frequently left much to be desired and they seldom approached the quality of care in the main hospital system: half had no operating theatre, less than one-quarter had an elevator, and they seldom had X-ray apparatus, laboratories or resident doctors.[61] *Lancet* described one such private hospital for the middle class which was located in a large London house. It was equipped with an operating room and 34 beds (12 in separate private rooms) and prices ranged from four to six guineas a week, but no mention was made of such things as X-ray rooms, pathology laboratories and other diagnostic facilities. As *Lancet* remarked, 'the prospectus . . . [gave] the impression of a moderately priced nursing home under medical supervision, with expert staff available at modified fees, [rather] than of a fully equipped modern hospital'.[62]

Predictably, arguments were frequently made that the poor were the most privileged in terms of access to the best care. An article in *The Hospital* entitled 'The Advantages of Poverty' claimed that the poor, as a result of their easy access to hospital care, could most easily secure the opinions of the best consultants. In contrast, wealthier sections of the population received only inferior care:

> Any arrangements that can possibly be made in a private house are at the best merely makeshift, while it is doubtful . . . if there is a single nursing home in existence in which conditions are not passed which, in a hospital, surgeons would absolutely condemn. The rich man

with all his wealth does not, and practically cannot, obtain the scientific advantage, which the poor man can and does obtain for nothing.[63]

Such sentiments were echoed by many others during the twenties and thirties. Periodically, the issue was raised as to how treatment should be provided for middle class patients. Should nursing homes be expanded and improved? Or should the middle class be admitted to voluntary and local hospitals? But with the exception of the patients in question, the latter solution was generally opposed, and the annexation of most middle class patients in a separate hospital system presented a dilemma which continued until the introduction of the NHS. The historical role of the hospitals in serving working class patients remained relatively unchanged until 1948.

National Health Insurance

The provision of primary medical care for working class patients during the late nineteenth century was deficient in several respects. Its quality was often doubtful and when patients were excluded from the schemes organised by friendly societies and medical clubs etc., they had no option but to rely on the overworked outpatient departments of the hospitals. But as the efficacy of medicine increased and 'an average patient treated by an average practitioner could expect a better than fifty-fifty chance of improvement',[64] a major change occurred in the provision of primary care for the working class which at least partially resolved some of these deficiencies. The introduction of the National Health Insurance scheme was the first major attempt on the part of the state to provide free general medical care to workers above the level of destitution and it laid the basis for the later development of a free health service. Coming into effect in 1913, the scheme provided primary medical care from general practitioners and sickness benefit to all manual workers and others who were paid £250 a year or less.[65] Insurance was covered by contributions of 4d. a week from employees, 3d. from employers, and 2d. from the Treasury — Lloyd George's 'ninepence for fourpence'. Whereas the local insurance committees were responsible for providing medical services, Approved Societies were responsible for providing workers with sick pay and for distributing other benefits which included dental treatment, hospital and convalescent care, medical and surgical appliances, and ophthalmic treatment.[66] These additional benefits were financed from the surplus held by each Approved Society after other expenses had been met.

While National Health Insurance was an important step towards a more comprehensive system of socialised medicine, it contained several anomalies. Approved Societies were not compelled to accept members and they generally refused membership to the chronic sick, but since additional benefits were only available through the societies, these patients received only the basic medical and cash benefits. Those most in need of care were least able to benefit from the scheme; they were unable to obtain dental treatment, hospital and convalescent care, medical and surgical appliances, and ophthalmic treatment. Even those workers who were accepted as members of Approved Societies faced problems in securing additional benefits. These benefits were financed from the surplus held by each society after other expenses had been met, and thus where demand for general practitioner care and sickness benefit was high, the surplus was small and few extra benefits could be financed. Where morbidity was high, where need was greatest, additional care was least available.

A further anomaly existed in that it was financially more advantageous for a worker to be drawing unemployment benefit than to be receiving sickness benefit. Writing in the late thirties, Herbert noted that an unemployed man with a wife and one child received 30s. per week in unemployment benefit if he was fit, whereas if he was unemployed due to sickness, he received 15s. in sickness benefit. He remarked that 'Doctors are often placed in the embarrassing position of being asked to sign off patients who should still be receiving medical attention solely in order that they may draw unemployment benefit.'[67]

There is also some evidence that the care received by panel patients under National Health Insurance was inferior to that available to fee paying patients.[68] The care and attention for such patients was claimed to be perfunctory — doctors were more interested in their more lucrative private patients and since these were financially the most important section of their practice, many doctors would employ an assistant to treat their panel patients while they devoted their own time to their private patients. If, on the other hand, a practice was made up solely of panel patients, the doctor's list was likely to be much larger than in a mixed practice. Though, in theory, panel patients were entitled to all necessary drugs free of charge, there were pressures on doctors to choose the cheapest: above average costs of prescribing were likely to be questioned and the doctor might even have to bear part of the excess cost himself. Doctors were, therefore, likely to err on the side of safety and restrict pharmaceutical benefits. This was not likely to be the case with private patients.

In such ways, the National Health Insurance scheme failed to meet many of the medical needs of workers. Those most in need of treatment and care generally had access to a limited number of benefits. While unemployment benefit was paid at higher rate than sickness benefit, there was a strong deterrent to seeking medical care. When care was sought, it was apparently inferior to that received by private patients. Moreover, the scheme was by no means self-supporting, even with respect to primary medical care; whereas the incentive for doctors had previously been to restrict the numbers of people treated at out-patient departments, so as to ensure themselves paying patients, now there was an incentive for doctors to reduce their workload, at least with respect to panel patients. They were paid on a *per capita* basis for these, and it was to their advantage to refer the more troublesome cases to hospital outpatient departments. Thus, the outpatient departments lost many of their more trivial cases, but retained the more trouble-some and time-consuming ones. In effect, they acquired a new role in complementing the work of the general practitioner by providing a specialist or consultative service. But despite the inadequacies of National Health Insurance, it was seen as an advance in the provision of medical care for the working class and while not uncritical, workers recognised the merits of the scheme and in later decades campaigned for its extension to their dependents.

The scheme did not provide coverage for children and women who were not engaged in paid labour. They, together with others not eligible for National Health Insurance benefits, continued to provide for their general medical needs through the outpatient departments of hospitals and through membership in friendly societies, family clubs, and provident medical associations. These latter were endorsed by the BMA, and seen by the medical profession as an effective solution to the problems of lay control experienced by doctors working in some form of contract practice. They were formed by doctors working in the same area who would share patients' contributions in proportion to the number of patients for which each was responsible. They were intended for lower income groups, people earning less than £250 per annum, and their membership grew steadily. Herbert notes that in the late thirties there were over 650,000 persons in sixty different societies, with the London service being extended to middle class families with incomes up to £550 per annum, and fees ranging from £4 to £5 per annum for a family of four.[69] For many, most particularly low income families, the main motive for joining such schemes was to avoid the need to rely on charity or public assistance. As the Royal Commission on the operation of the National Health Insurance scheme indicated:

> There is a certain amount of evidence that many insured persons are reluctant to go to outpatients' departments, as a charity, while they would not hesitate to avail themselves of the same specialist services if included in medical benefit, as they would then feel that they had a full, legal, and moral right to receive the services when needed.[70]

Conclusion

Common assumptions about the introduction of social welfare legislation lead us to expect that before the introduction of the NHS, the poor and working class were either denied the care available to middle class patients, or that the care which they received was of distinctly lesser quality than that obtained by middle class patients. However, it appears that no such simple statements can be made concerning class inequalities in access to care and use of health services prior to 1948. Free public and charitable care was available for the working class even in the mid-nineteenth century and treatment was provided at small cost through various types of contributory schemes. From 1911, workers received free general practitioner care under National Health Insurance, while their dependents continued to receive treatment from the same sources as previously. The rising costs of care led to limitations being placed on the amount of free care available, and those above the level of destitution began to be charged for a part of the cost of treatment, yet these increasing costs were partly balanced by the rapid growth in membership of contributory schemes serving working class patients. However, middle class patients were generally excluded from membership in such schemes and, by paying high private fees, they helped to subsidise the care of working class patients: they received few financial concessions in obtaining care. There is little data to indicate the use made of health services by patients of different class, but that which is available for the two years before the introduction of the NHS give no clear indication of lower rates of consultation with doctors on the part of working class patients.[71]

Differences in the quality of care received by working class and middle class patients were probably minimal in the mid-nineteenth century, as care was uniformly quite poor. But as medical care increased in sophistication, it is possible that in terms of general practitioner care, middle class patients received better treatment. Yet this was not so with respect to hospital care. In the early 1940s, local and voluntary hospitals were still admitting mainly working class patients while middle class patients were generally confined to the smaller and less well equipped private hospital system. In this respect — and in the fact that they received no financial concessions in obtaining care — middle class patients were in a disadvantaged position. It is not that problems in obtaining health care were non-existent for working class families — even small costs may have severely strained the purses of workers' families, and the moral stigma of accepting charity may have inhibited some from obtaining care. But it is inappropriate to recognise problems as existing for the working class alone; the traditional organisation of health services posed considerable problems for middle class families also. Not until the introduction of the NHS were these problems resolved.

Notes

1. This discussion of sources of medical care in the mid-nineteenth century is largely based on M. Bruce, *The Coming of the Welfare State* (B.T. Batsford, London, 1966); B. Abel-Smith, *The Hospitals 1800-1948* (Heinemann, London, 1964); B. Webb and S. Webb, *The State and the Doctor* (Longmans, Green and Company, London, 1910); Ruth G. Hodgkinson, *The Origins of the National Health Service* (The Wellcome Historical Medical Library, London, 1967).

2. S.W.F. Holloway, 'Medical Education in England, 1830-1858: A Sociological Analysis', *History*, vol. 49 (October, 1964), p. 316.

3. Abel-Smith, *The Hospitals 1800-1948*, p. 1; Hodgkinson, *The Origins of the National Health Service*, p. 593.

4. Rodney M. Coe, *Sociology of Medicine* (McGraw-Hill, London, 1970), p. 245.

5. P.H.J.H. Gosden, *The Friendly Societies in England* (Manchester University Press, Manchester, 1961).

6. Ibid., p. 7.

7. Bruce, *The Coming of the Welfare State*, p. 96; Royal Commission on the Poor Laws and Relief of Distress, vol. 1, *Report* (HMSO, London, 1909), p. 333.

8. This is emphasised by the fact that the decision to grant an order was made by a non-medical officer on the basis of non-medical circumstances — destitution.

9. Webb and Webb, *State and Doctor*, p. 48.

10. Hodgkinson *The Origins of the National Health Service*, p. 695.

11. S. Webb and B. Webb (eds.), *The Break-up of the Poor Law* (Longmans, Green and Company, London, 1909), p. 219.

12. S. Leff, *The Health of the People* (Victor Gollancz, London, 1950), p. 65.

13. Webb and Webb, *State and Doctor*, pp. 42-3.

14. Ibid., p. 52.

15. McKeown and Lowe argue that medicine had relatively little impact on health until the second quarter of the twentieth century. Until then, environmental factors were largely responsible for improvements in health. T. McKeown and C.R. Lowe, *An Introduction to Social Medicine*, 2nd edn (Blackwell, Oxford, 1974), pp. 3-22.

16. Abel-Smith, *The Hospitals 1800-1948*, p. 2.

17. I am assuming that medicine gradually became more effective and that the

use of health services became one important determinant of people's mortality and morbidity experience. Equality of access to medical care is thus an important element in achieving a reduction of inequalities in health. Though common, these assumptions are, however, open to question. For one challenging discussion of the impact of medicine see Ivan Illich, *Limits to Medicine* (McClelland and Stewart, Toronto, 1976).

18. For an analysis of changing attitudes towards health see Holloway, 'Medical Education in England, 1830-1858: A Sociological Analysis.'

19. R. Bendix, *Work and Authority in Industry* (Harper and Row, New York, 1963), pp. 109-16.

20. Holloway, 'Medical Education in England, 1830-1858: A Sociological Analysis', p. 320.

21. Ibid., p. 320.

22. Abel-Smith, *The Hospitals 1800-1948*, p. 85; Webb and Webb, *State and Doctor*, Ch. 3.

23. Abel-Smith, *The Hospitals 1800-1948*, pp. 130-1; Leff, *The Health of the People*, p. 99.

24. Webb and Webb, *State and Doctor*, p. 123.

25. Abel-Smith, *The Hospitals 1800-1948*, pp. 122-5.

26. Royal Commission on the Poor Laws, p. 328.

27. Ibid., p. 329.

28. Ibid., p. 330.

29. The Local Government Act of 1929 allowed local authorities to appropriate Poor Law institutions, but even in 1937, the majority of sick beds were still operated under the Poor Law. Abel-Smith, *The Hospitals 1800-1948*, p. 371; S.M. Herbert, *Britain's Health* (Penguin, Harmondsworth, 1939), p. 122-3.

30. Abel-Smith, *The Hospitals 1800-1948*, p. 296.

31. Ibid., p. 309.

32. A. Lindsey, *Socialized Medicine in England and Wales* (University of North Carolina Press, Chapel Hill, NC, 1962), p. 15.

33. Abel-Smith, *The Hospitals 1800-1948*, p. 327.

34. Ibid., p. 332.

35. Ibid., p. 386.

36. Herbert, *Britain's Health*, p. 102.

37. Abel-Smith, *The Hospitals 1800-1948*, p. 149.

38. *Lancet*, ii (1927), p. 1277.

39. Ibid., p. 1277.

40. Ibid., i (1927), p. 270.

41. Ibid., ii (1928), p. 175.

42. King Edward's Hospital Fund for London, *Provision for the Professional and Middle Classes at Voluntary Hospitals in London* (Kind Edward's Hospital Fund for London, London, 1936), p. 4.

43. *Lancet*, i (1934), p. 792.

44. Ibid., p. 793.

45. Ibid., ii (1934), p. 1402.

46. Ibid., i (1934),p. 793.

47. King Edward's Hospital Fund for London, p. 4.

48. *Lancet*, ii (1934), p.811.

49. Ibid., p. 962.

50. Ibid., p. 1210.

51. Nuffield Provincial Hospitals Trust, *The Hospital Surveys: The Domesday Book of the Hospital Services* (Oxford University Press, London, 1946).

52. *Lancet*, ii (1927), p. 1278.

53. Ibid., ii (1928), p. 175.

54. Ibid., i (1932), p. 1180.
55. Ibid., i (1934), pp. 770, 820.
56. Ibid., i (1932),pp. 1327.
57. Ibid., i (1927), p. 269.
58. Ibid., p. 665.
59. Abel-Smith, *The Hospitals 1800-1948*, p. 339.
60. Ibid., p. 343.
61. Ibid., p. 343.
62. *Lancet*, i (1927), p. 665.
63. Abel-Smith, *The Hospitals 1800-1948*, p. 192.
64. Eliot Friedson, *Profession of Medicine: A Study of the Sociology of Applied Knowledge* (Harper and Row, New York, 1970), p. 16.
65. The limit was raised to £420 in January 1942. A thorough discussion of National Health Insurance can be found in H. Levy, *National Health Insurance* (Cambridge University Press, Cambridge, 1944).
66. Any group could register as an Approved Society as long as it was non-profit making and democratically organised. Friendly societies, trade unions and life assurance companies eagerly took on such a role, where necessary, creating non-profit sections. For them, it was an introduction to potential members and clients who might be persuaded to take advantage of other services they had to offer.
67. Herbert, *Britain's Health*, p. 98.
68. Yet the Royal Commission investigating the operation of National Health Insurance, concluded that panel patients did not receive inferior care. Royal Commission on National Health Insurance, *Report* (HMSO, London, 1926).
69. Herbert, *Britain's Health*, p. 74.
70. Levy, *National Health Insurance*, p. 164.
71. Class differences in rates of consultation are discussed in Ch. 6.

3 FINANCIAL AND ORGANISATIONAL PROBLEMS WITHIN THE HEALTH SECTOR

In seeking to understand the introduction of the NHS, it is important that we look beyond the problems in access to health care which were experienced by patients of different social class. Not only is it inappropriate to emphasise the barriers to care which existed for working class patients, it is also too limiting to focus simply on the issue of access to care. For despite the fact that both working class and middle class patients experienced difficulties in obtaining adequate medical care, this does not appear to be the main reason for the introduction of the NHS. Inadequacies in the organisation and coverage of National Health Insurance and the relative exclusion of middle class patients from the best hospital care and from insurance schemes were not trivial problems, but there were many other organisational and financial problems which also demanded attention. Rather than being a response to class conflict and the disadvantages experienced by working class patients, it appears that the NHS was introduced in order to rationalise the organisation and delivery of health care and to create a stable financial base within the health sector. Though several writers have stressed the importance of class conflict in explaining the growth of social welfare legislation,[1] in this instance it is more fitting to recognise that the state was responding to the organisational and financial problems which plagued the health services. These became increasingly severe during the twenties and thirties and much of the debate over reform, as well as governments' explanations of the need for a national health service, focused on the necessity of rationalising the organisation and financing of health care. In later chapters we will look at the ways in which representatives of the organised working class, the medical profession and the state defined the inadequacies of the health care system. For the moment, let us focus on the wide range of problems which existed; these prompted a recognition of a need for change and structured a situation in which the NHS could be introduced.

The Emerging Crisis in the Hospital System

The increasing costs of new medical technologies, of new diagnostic procedures and of more specialised personnel were a source of financial pressure for both voluntary and public hospitals.[2] The early growth of specialisation is evident in the clinics opened by the larger teaching hospitals: Guy's Hospital introduced a clinic for skin diseases in 1851 and for aural diseases in 1862; in 1867, St Bartholomew's Hospital started an ophthalmology department and by 1880, it had clinics for diseases of throat and skin, for orthopaedics, obstetrics and gynaecology; and the London Hospital opened an obstetrics department in 1852, an ear, nose and throat department in 1866, and were specialising in orthopaedics also by 1875.[3] By the 1940s, many hospitals which had at one time employed a few consultants together with a small nursing and administrative staff, employed a wide range of specialists. Apart from more specialised consultants, laboratory technicians, dieticians, occupational therapists, radiographers and many others had become part of the changing hospital system. In addition to the increasing costs of employing these more specialised personnel, rising wages further strained hospital budgets. For example, the wages of nursing staff rose substantially during World War I; the pay of personnel in military hospitals was relatively high and with the advent of the war, personnel in civilian hospitals received pay increases to bring wages to a similar level. The Local Government Board revised the scale of pay for nursing staff in institutions used in the war effort, so that they received about 3 per cent more than nurses in Poor Law instititutions. Soon after, the voluntary hospitals and Poor Law institutions followed suit in order to maintain competitive wages. In the Sheffield Royal Infirmary, for example, the annual wages of probationer nurses rose from £5 in 1914 to £30 in 1918, while those for sisters rose from £30 to £40-50 a year in the same period.[4] In 1891, salaries and wages accounted for 26.9 per cent of the ordinary expenditure of selected London voluntary hospitals and by 1938 the proportion had risen to 38.5 per cent. In the provinces, voluntary hospitals saw an increase from 24.2 per cent to 37.8 per cent over the same period.[5]

As well as increasing the number and diversity of the new personnel employed, the rapid developments in medical knowledge also increased the costs of diagnosis and treatment. Not only did discoveries follow each other in rapid succession, broader and broader applications were also developed for these. In 1918, one major provincial hospital conducted less than six hundred X-ray examinations, but by the late 1940s, it was performing nearly 20,000. In the same hospital, the number of pathological examinations in 1947 was thirty-three times the number in 1927. And the same period saw a fifty-fold increase in blood counts.[6] Such increases in the use of diagnostic techniques also played a part in the escalation of the operating costs of hospitals.

Unlike business concerns, the growth of the hospitals could lead simply to a growth in spending capacity and not necessarily to a greater earning capacity. The expenditure per bed in selected London and provincial voluntary hospitals almost doubled between 1891 and 1938 — an increase from £65.60 to £121 at 1914 prices. Total expenditure rose from £1,102 to £16,469 during this period and salaries and wages became the largest item of expenditure in the London hospitals after 1891, and in the provinces, after 1911.[7] These increases in expenditure were aggravated by the fact that the majority of hospitals were of an uneconomic size; of roughly seven hundred 'all purpose' voluntary hospitals, at least five hundred had less than 100 beds and about half of these had less than 30 beds.[8] The smaller hospitals were most likely to be located in the provinces:

Before the war there were, in all, 49 voluntary hospitals in South Wales and Monmouthshire of which 5 had over 100 beds, 21 had 31-100 beds and 23 had less than 30 beds. In Berkshire, Buckinghamshire and Oxfordshire there were 75 hospitals of all types (voluntary and municipal), 41 of which had less than 50 beds. In addition, there were 89 private nursing homes with an average of less than nine beds apiece.[9]

The hospitals might have tackled their financial problems by merging expanding, or simply by co-ordinating their activities, but adequate co-ordination was never achieved, few mergers occurred, and most hospitals were prevented from expanding due either to a lack of capital or the fact that adjacent land was just not available.[10]

Financial pressures were particularly problematic for the voluntary hospitals. The charitable donations on which they depended were not falling, but neither were they increasing apace with rising expenditures and though philanthropy might finance a new ward or a new operating theatre, it did not necessarily provide funds for the continuing operation of these. The hospital system had grown in response to donations and legacies rather than a demonstrated need for services and thus some areas had too many hospitals, others, too few; some were relatively affluent, others operated with a continuing deficit. The philanthropic base of the hospitals had led to haphazard growth and had failed to provide a stable source of support for operation and maintenance expenditures. It was difficult to view the future with optimism, for the increasing burden of taxation represented a forced charity and foreshadowed a decline or stabilisation of voluntary contributions.

The late 1800s and early 1900s were marked by intermittent
financial crises within the voluntary hospital system. In 1887, the total
deficit of teaching hospitals was over £32,000. Three years later it had
risen to about £100,000 and in 1889 it was claimed that 2,000 beds in
London were closed due to lack of funds.[11] But the onset of war
helped the hospitals. The voluntary hospitals which were important for
the war effort were paid £880,000 by the War Office between 1914 and
1919 — to cover the costs of care for the sick and wounded. It was
claimed that this amount fell short of actual costs by about £530,000,
but charitable donations, prompted by heightened social conscience,
increased during this period and for some hospitals, more than compen-
sated for their deficits. Between 1915 and 1919 charitable organisations held a surplus in excess of £7,000,000.[12] But the gains were
temporary and the effect of post war inflation was such as to place the
hopitals in another critical financial situation. By 1920 they were once
again in financial straits; 452 provincial hospitals shared a total deficit
of £280,000 and 113 Metropolitan hospitals reported a combined
deficit of £370,000.[13] The Manchester Royal Infirmary reported that it
needed £9,000 extra each year to restore the finances of the hospital,
the London Fever Hospital was said to be closing, and the National
Hospital was discharging all of its patients.[14]

Grants from the King Edward Hospital Fund and the National
Relief Fund helped the hospitals meet their deficits and the crisis was
averted. Yet it was recognised that this was no more than a temporary
solution. In 1921, the Cave Committee was appointed to investigate the
financial situation of the voluntary hospitals and it recommended
among other things, that the hospitals receive temporary support from
the government for a period of two years, while they improved their
financial base. The idea of temporary support was a measure designed
to avert the immediate crisis without compromising the independence
of the hospitals, but though the Committee recommended the sum of
£1,000,000, the government gave only half this amount. The accounts
of the hospitals were restored to a momentary state of health and by
1923, 624 provincial hospitals were operating with a surplus of
£270,000 and 116 Metropolitan hospitals had a total surplus of
£230,000.[15] But a more permanent solution to the problem was
obviously necessary.

The Cave Committee had expressed optimism about the future of
the voluntary hospital system, yet only if it utilised additional sources
of revenue. Several sources of revenue did, in fact, become increasingly
important during the twenties and thirties, but the optimism of the

Committee was unjustified for these were successful only as temporary measures and none provided the hospitals with adequate financial support. One strategy which the Committee had recommended was that of securing contributions from Approved Societies towards the cost of care of their members, and some hospitals were successful in obtaining such contributions. In addition, almoners were more rigorously checking whether patients could afford to pay towards the costs of their care and many hospitals opened small private wings for patients who paid between three and seven guineas a week for their beds. But such provision was never very extensive and the President of the British Medical Association (BMA), notwithstanding the Association's opposition to pay beds in hospitals, could argue in 1927 that the scale of provision was 'utterly and grotesquely inadequate'.[16]

It was an existing source of revenue which became increasingly important and which rescued many hospitals from financial straits; hospital contributory schemes. In these, members paid small weekly contributions towards the future costs of hospital care, and, in many cases, employers added a portion of the contribution. The membership of these schemes increased during the twenties as working class patients sought to provide for the day when they would need hospital care, and when they wished to avoid undergoing means tests. The Hospital Savings Association — the largest of such schemes — reported an increase in membership from 62,390 in 1924, to 351,865 three years later[17] and to 650,000 in 1929.[18] The Liverpool Workpeople's Hospital Fund claimed a membership of 65,000 in its first six months of operation,[19] and in its first two months the Birmingham Contributory Scheme reported that nearly 1,000 firms had joined and almost 250,000 workingmen had been enrolled.[20] In 1927, the President of the BMA, in an address on 'The Voluntary Hospital and its Future' remarked that 'the income derived from the various kinds of contributory schemes is now double that of any of the four principal items of income'.[21]

Such new sources of revenue represented larger and larger portions of the current income of voluntary hospitals. Pinker's study of the income and expenditure of selected voluntary hospitals does not present income from contributory schemes, from Approved Societies and from private patients as separate categories, but it does show that receipts for services rendered became the single most important source of income by 1921 in the provinces and by 1938 in London. Patients' payments and workingmen's contributions accounted for 8.3 per cent of income for selected voluntary hospitals in England and Wales in

1891, 15.9 per cent in 1911, 38.1 per cent in 1921 and 52.1 per cent in 1938. The proportion of income derived from voluntary gifts and investments declined over the same period; from 87.5 per cent in 1891 to 39.5 per cent in 1938.[22] Voluntary contributions were not declining in amount, they simply represented a lessening portion of hospital income. The Annual Statistical Review of the King Edward's Hospital Fund for London for 1931 indicated that the depression did not have an adverse effect on charitable donations to voluntary hospitals. The total income of 142 London hospitals was £3,811,000 (£34,000 more than in 1930) and they reported an aggregate surplus of £76,000 (£4,000 less than in the previous year). The number of hospitals with a surplus rose from seventy-two to eighty-five, a fact interpreted as a 'substantial advance' towards individual solvency; a decline in subscriptions and donations had been expected 'but a happy fate stepped in to make this loss more than good by implanting "holy and wholesome thoughts" into the minds of testators'.[23] But it was noted that such donations were bound to be an uncertain quantity in the future, and that the new revenue sources were increasingly important:

> Contributory schemes are increasing in number and importance, and patients generally are learning that, in so far as they are able, it is their duty to make a practical return for what is done for them. Meanwhile the 'pay-bed' is making its contribution at once to a growing necessity and to the solvency of the voluntary hospitals.[24]

Yet neither could these new sources of income be relied upon to prevent future crises. Given the opposition of the BMA, the hospitals' wish to avoid jeopardising appeals to charity, and the fact that many· trusts were tied to the provision of charitable care rather than financing private treatment, the growth in the number of beds for private patients was obviously limited. While contributory schemes added considerably to hospital revenues, they were still inadequate for many hospitals, and these, unable to meet the costs of improvements, expansion of facilities and even operating costs, continued to face intermittent crises. In 1927, Swansea Hospital was in a serious financial position, having almost exhausted its overdraft limit of £60,000. It was noted that 'unless means are found of increasing its revenue, there will be no alternative but to close portions of the hospital and bring monthly expenditure into line with monthly revenue'.[25] Yet despite this critical situation, the governors of the hospital decided 'not to admit or assist with advice or treatment any person who is able to pay fully for the same'.[26] On the

other hand, the Royal Northern Hospital, carrying a debt of over
£81,000, was in 1928 considering the practicability of providing a
separate block of wards for middle class patients.[27] The contributory
scheme of the Birmingham and Midland Ear and Throat Hospital was
its chief source of income in 1931, but the resources of the hospital
were 'quite unequal to cope with the work' and an up-to-date building
was declared to be imperative.[28]

In 1936 the King's Fund reported a net aggregate deficit (of
£64,000) for the first time since 1926. The Fund was hoping to maintain the annual distribution of £300,000 to hospitals in its area, but in
order for this to continue, the treasurer noted that:

> there must be a substantial increase in income . . . Until 1934,
> current receipts provided the amount required. In 1935, however,
> there was a shortage of nearly £7,000 and in 1936 another shortage
> of over £7,000. But for some exceptional income from investments
> during the year the deficit would have been very much larger. For
> eight years legacies had remained very steady at between £60,000
> and £70,000 a year, but in 1936 they had amounted to only
> £44,000.[29]

Yet despite the success of the Fund in maintaining its payments to the
hospitals, 59 of 145 London voluntary hospitals ended the year with a
deficit. While *Lancet* summarised the position of the hospitals and the
role of the King's Fund in positive terms, it was hardly a description of
a financially healthy hospital system: 'The vitality of the voluntary
hospitals is remarkable. Their final financial submersion, both individu-
ally and collectively, is annually predicted, but they keep rising to the
surface, like the cat with nine lives.'[30]

As a consequence of the financial pressures under which most hospitals operated, they were often poorly equipped, under-staffed and
housed in quite inadequate old buildings. Referring to the Hospital
Surveys which reported on the situation of the hospitals in 1938,
Titmuss writes that 'one report after another spoke of large old-
fashioned wards, out-of-date kitchens, poor and insufficient equipment,
inadequate or non-existing laboratories, ugly and prison-like buildings
and old dilapidated structures'.[31] Even the more prestigious teaching
hospitals were often either unsafe or quite antiquated.[32] But there were
wide variations between hospitals — some operated for long periods
with no serious deficit, others were in a state of almost continual financial crisis. In the quality of their medical and nursing staff, their

standards of work and the range of equipment and diagnostic and treatment facilities they were quite diverse. But though world renowned teaching hospitals seemed to share little in common with tiny cottage hospitals, they were alike in their financial struggle to maintain themselves.

It was World War II which most clearly demonstrated the need for reform. Until this time little information on the hospital system had been collected, but in the urgent preparations for the Emergency Medical Service, the inadequacy of the hospital system, even for peacetime purposes, became obvious. Specialists who left the familiar environment of the well-provided metropolitan and teaching hospitals to work in local hospitals which were, in contrast, often small and poorly equipped, became much more aware of the serious deficiencies in the hospital service.

Quite apart from broader organisational problems, the precarious financial base of the voluntary hospitals was more clearly recognised and a stable and continuing source of revenue was seen to be essential. Many of these hospitals were damaged in air raids, others had found it necessary to postpone renovation and expansion projects and, despite the fact that they ended the war with added reserves of over £10,000,000, they were not in a strong financial position. Prices were increasing again while interest rates were low and if the standards of war time service were to be maintained, the hospitals needed an additional source of income.[33] No strong private interests had become involved in the hospital services, and it was to the state alone that the hospitals could turn for the continuing financial support they needed. They had already benefited from public payments during the war and pre-war period and thus precedents for state support had been established. In 1920, Lord Knutsford, Chairman of the London Hospital, had suggested that state aid was imperative to ensure the continuation of the voluntary hospitals, and that such aid should cover one-third of hospital expenditures.[34] At that time, the idea was dismissed by many people as it was seen to threaten the independence of the voluntary hospital system, but by the forties it was generally recognised that more formal ties must be established between the hospitals and the state, with the latter providing something more than intermittent grants to avert crises. It was the precise form of the relationship between the state and the voluntary hospitals which was open to question; the hospitals sought to preserve their autonomy despite public financing; others valued this autonomy less highly.

Problems of Distribution and Co-ordination of Services

The financial problems which confronted the voluntary hospitals were linked with fundamental organisational problems within the health services. There was almost no organised national system of health services — even National Health Insurance was administered through locally based Approved Societies. Medical care was available from a wide variety of sources, almost all of which were local in character; primary care might be obtained through National Health Insurance, a friendly society, doctors' clubs, some form of contract practice, from private practitioners or from the outpatient departments of voluntary or public hospitals. Inpatient care could be obtained from any one of a number of different types of hospitals — public, voluntary, cottage, home hospitals or private nursing homes. Apart from National Health Insurance coverage, people might either pay the full costs of care, belong to one or more of over three hundred local contributory schemes, or else receive free care. There was minimal co-ordination between these many and varied units responsible for providing and financing care and as a result, services were often wastefully duplicated, unevenly distributed and wide variations existed in the standard of care provided. As the provision of medical services expanded and the health system increased in complexity and required greater capital investment as a result of new medical technology, these problems became more severe and more obvious, and a need to rationalise the system was more and more frequently recognised.

One major problem was that of the uneven distribution of facilities and manpower. Quite apart from a general shortage of hospital beds (it was estimated that the supply of beds was one-third below the desired minimum), hospital provision varied from one area to another. The voluntary hospital system had grown in haphazard fashion — in response to donations and legacies — and the most plentiful provision of beds was in the larger industrial centres. Local authorities were enabled rather than required to provide hospital facilities and the quality and number of these facilities were quite uneven, since the attitudes of local councillors varied, as also did the size and resources of the authorities. In the London region there were 10.2 beds per 1,000 population, while in South Wales the corresponding figure was 4.9, and in the Sheffield and East Midlands region, 5.1. Not only was there such variation between the areas, great disparities also existed within areas. For example, in the Yorkshire region there were 6.6 beds per 1,000 population, but this was an average of variations from 12.3 beds per 1,000 in Dewsbury and 10.8 in Halifax, to 4.9 beds in York and 3.1 in the North

Riding.[35]

The quality and provision of physician care also varied quite widely between areas. The distribution of consultants paralleled that of the larger and more prestigious teaching hospitals and a third of qualified specialists were located in London.[36]

> Before the war some counties were without a single gynaecologist; the Eastern counties had no thoracic surgeons, dermatologists and paediatricians and only two hospitals with psychiatrists on their staff; in South Wales and Monmouthshire only five out of 56 acute general and acute special hospitals had specialists in continuous charge of patients; in the Sheffield and East Midlands are a covering a population of 4,000,000 'paediatrics is a relatively undeveloped subject', plastic surgery was not organised at all, while less than six doctors restricted their work to the administration of anaesthetics.[37]

Public hospitals found it difficult to attract the better specialists and certain areas were served only by visiting consultants. Cottage hospitals were staffed by general practitioners and specialists were called in only for very complex cases. In some towns, specialists combined general practice with part time specialisation and since this was one of the least desirable conditions of practice, it tended to attract the least able.[38] As a consequence, some of the worst medical care was provided in rural areas, where local general practitioners did surgery beyond their competence and in the absence of adequate support staff and equipment. Referring to such areas starved of consultants, one of the Hospital Surveys pointed out that:

> In the past the tendency has been for the general practitioner gradually to drift into surgery, or whatever branch of medicine he is most interested in, and to do this as an off-shoot from his general practice; he may be entirely self-taught and without proper training for the particular branch he chooses.[39]

Other staff were under pressure to become 'jacks of all trades'; in many of the smaller hospitals 'the matron was expected to act as the radiographer, to carry out the work of almoner, and to be midwife and cook, in addition to her work as matron.[40]

General practitioners were also unevenly distributed throughout the country. Understandably perhaps, doctors preferred to locate in middle class urban areas, thus avoiding the isolation of rural practice and the lesser autonomy of the various forms of contract practice which served working class areas. Instead, they preferred the autonomy, higher fees and more congenial working conditions associated with private practice. Quite obviously many were not able to achieve such an ideal, but the distribution of doctors did reflect such preferences. Middle class areas were likely to have a surfeit of general practitioners while working class areas needed to attract more doctors. In the late thirties, there were 50 per cent less doctors *per capita* in South Wales as in London, and only 25 per cent as many *per capita* in the industrial Midlands as in Bournemouth.[41] Hastings had one doctor per 1,178 population, Swindon one for every 3,100, Greenock one per 3,500 and South Shields one per 4,100.[42]

These problems of maldistribution, inadequate financing and shortages of personnel and facilities were intensified by the fact that there was minimal co-ordination between the myriad units providing and financing care. For example, the relationship between the two main hospital systems was marked by jealousy and rivalry and the links which existed between them occurred on an *ad hoc* basis; by making contributions to a voluntary hospital and thus having a claim on its services, a public hospital might be represented on the Board, or a Medical Officer of Health might be appointed to the staff of a voluntary hospital. But few formal ties were established. Yet neither was there much co-ordination of activities within each of the hospital systems. The hospitals generally had parochial allegiances and were unwilling to co-operate in new projects or in co-ordinating the types of services they provided. The Hospital Survey of the Sheffield and East Midlands region pointed out one such instance:

> The bad results of strict adherence to existing local government
> boundaries are nowhere better exemplified than in Leicestershire
> and Nottinghamshire, where the respective Counties and County
> Boroughs have each erected good modern sanatoria each pair being
> only 5 miles apart, instead of combining to produce more efficient
> and larger hospital units.[43]

In 1922 the Cave Committee had noted the lack of co-ordination and consequent inefficiency of the voluntary hospitals, but this improved little during the twenties and thirties. The King Edward's Hospital Fund for London, which had been in existence since 1897, had sought to rationalise and co-ordinate the activities of those hospitals within its area and grants which it made to individual hospitals were often conditional upon hospitals merging or using funds for specified purposes. The efforts of the Fund do not appear to have been particularly successful, though as Abel-Smith argues, it probably prevented a further deterioration of the situation. Other efforts at co-ordination were similarly ineffectual. For example, the Liverpool General Hospitals' Co-ordination Committee was formed in 1932 to 'secure better co-operation among the 22 voluntary hospitals of the city'[44] but its likelihood of success was small since the committee was 'purely advisory, with no power of executive action, but with power to publish its conclusions'.[45] Also, in 1932, the London Voluntary Hospitals' Committee and the Central Public Health Committee of the London County Council announced their intention to collaborate in a survey of the medical, surgical and ancillary services in the county. Without such information, it was claimed, 'the best use cannot be made of the facilities provided by each system, overlapping cannot be avoided, and economical effective progress is impossible'.[46] In 1935 the British Hospitals' Association appointed the Voluntary Hospitals' Commission to enquire into the financial and organisational problems of the hospitals and to make recommendations for change. The Commission reported in 1937 and, among other things, recommended local co-ordination, strong regional and central organisation and the creation of regional funds similar to the King Edward's Hospital Fund for London, but the war prevented any action which might have been taken on its proposals.[47] Despite such attempts to achieve co-ordination, the Hospital Surveys concluded that: 'In no area is there a genuine pooling of facilities in an attempt to extract from the combined resources the maximum advantage to the population.'[48]

Even at the outbreak of war, there was an appalling ignorance about the health system.[49] It was not until the Hospital Surveys were completed in 1946 that a reasonably accurate picture of hospital resources was available.[50] Proposals for change and critiques of the health services which were published during the inter-war years were not based on extensive and systematically collected data. An awareness of the financial and organisational problems had emerged largely from the day-to-day experience of those using or working within the health services, and the war both intensified these problems and heightened people's awareness of a need to rationalise the financing, organisation and delivery of health care. In hindsight, the situation was much worse than supposed, but nevertheless, a need for reform of the health system was quite widely recognised.

Conclusion

It is evident that the health services in England and Wales were
deficient in several respects. Working class and middle class patients
were, in different ways, disadvantaged in their access to medical care;
the National Health Insurance scheme was full of anomalies; hospitals
were inadequately financed and the revenue base of the voluntary
hospitals was quite insecure; hospital and physician services were
unevenly distributed throughout the country; and while many different
units were responsible for providing and financing care, there was
minimal co-ordination between these. Those studies which view the
NHS as a response to class conflict have focused on the barriers which
working class patients faced in obtaining health care. Clearly, this was
but one of several problems which can be identified within the health
sector. It is important that we recognise the broader range of organisational and financial problems, for in these lay the preconditions for
change. They provided the objective basis for pressures for reform and
structured a situation in which changes could be introduced.

But irrespective of the objective problems which existed within
the health services, what deficiencies were actually being identified
during the inter-war years? And by whom? To what extent was the
identification of problems translated into pressures for reform? What
types of changes were people proposing? Despite the fact that the
working cass was not singularly disadvantaged in access to care, and
even though a range of problems existed within the health services,
were representatives of the working class successful in shaping the
debate over reform? Did they succeed in creating a concern with the
problems faced by working class families and a belief in the desirability of some form of socialised medicine?

Notes

1. Frances Fox Pivan and Richard A. Cloward, *Regulating the Poor: The
Functions of Public Welfare* (Pantheon Books, New York, 1971); R. Miliband,
The State in Capitalist Society (Quartet, London, 1969); Vicente Navarro, *Class
Struggle, The State and Medicine* (Martin Robertson, London, 1978); J. Strachey,
Contemporary Capitalism (Victor Gollancz, London, 1956); Dorthy Wedderburn
(ed.), *Poverty, Inequality and Class Structure* (Cambridge University Press,
London, 1974).

2. This discussion of the hospitals relies heavily on B. Abel-Smith, *The
Hospitals 1800-1948* (Heinemann, London, 1964).

3. Ibid., p. 159.

4. Ibid., p. 269.

5. Robert Pinker, *English Hospital Statistics 1861-1938* (Heinemann, London, 1966), p. 157.

6. A. Lindsey, *Socialized Medicine in England and Wales* (University of North Carolina Press, Chapel Hill, NC, 1962), p. 24.

7. Pinker, *English Hospital Statistics 1861-1938*, pp. 154-8.

8. Harry Eckstein, *The English Health Service: Its Origins, Structure and Achievements* (Harvard University Press, Cambridge, Mass., 1958), p. 63.

9. Richard M. Titmuss, *Problems of Social Policy* (HMSO, London, 1976), p. 67.

10. Eckstein, *The English Health Service*, p. 64.

11. Abel-Smith, *The Hospitals 1800-1948*, p. 163.

12. Ibid., p. 282.

13. Ibid., p. 326.

14. Ibid., p.297.

15. Ibid., p. 326.

16. *Lancet*, i (1927), p. 270.

17. Ibid., i (1928), p. 634.

18. Abel-Smith, *The Hospitals 1800-1948*, p. 327.

19. *Lancet*, i (1928) p. 516.

20. Ibid., p. 529.

21. Ibid., i (1927), p. 270.

22. Pinker, *English Hospital Statistics 1861-1938*, p. 152.

23. *Lancet*, ii (1932), p. 324.

24. Ibid.

25. Ibid., ii (1927), p. 543.

26. Ibid., p. 909.

27. Ibid., i (1928), p. 727.

28. Ibid., i (1932), p. 1103.

29. Ibid., ii (1937), p. 38.

30. Ibid., p. 1444.

31. Titmuss, *Social Policy*, pp. 69-70.

32. Ibid., p. 65.

33. Abel-Smith, *The Hospitals 1800-1948*, p. 438.

34. Ibid., p. 296.

35. Eckstein, *The English Health Service*, pp. 57-8.

36. Abel-Smith, *The Hospitals 1800-1948*, p. 406.

37. Titmuss, *Social Policy*, p. 71, n. 1.

38. Eckstein, *The English Health Service*, p. 59.

39. Nuffield Provincial Hospitals Trust, *The Hospital Surveys: The Domesday Book of the Hospital Services* (University Press, Oxford, 1946), p. 10.

40. Titmuss, *Social Policy*, p. 67, n. 1.

41. Lindsey, *Socialized Medicine*, p. 7.

42. S. Leff, *The Health of the People* (Victor Gollancz, London, 1950), p. 210.

43. Nuffield Provincial Hospitals Trust, *The Hospital Surveys*, p. 14.

44. *Lancet*, ii (1932), p. 374.

45. Ibid.

46. Ibid., i (1932), p. 1008.

47. Abel-Smith, *The Hospitals 1800-1948*, pp. 412-23.

48. Nuffield Provincial Hospitals Trust, *The Hospital Surveys*, p. 15.

49. Titmuss, *Social Policy*, p. 164.

50. Ibid., p. 505.

4 WORKING CLASS PRESSURES FOR REFORM

The range of problems within the health services does, in itself, suggest that the NHS was not simply a response to demands for change from the working class. Yet the introduction of the service has often been explained in terms of the supposed radicalisation of the working class. For example, Navarro sees social legislation as flowing from an interplay of the social demands of labour and the social needs of capital and he argues that the concern with reform of the health services during the thirties and forties was in a large part a response to the radicalisation of the working class — radicalisation which prompted a defensive reaction on the part of the medical profession and the state.[1] Thus he sees the NHS as a response to the threat of a socialist alternative and an effort to secure the loyalty of the working class during war time. It may be the case that, despite other problems, representatives of the organised working class shaped the debate over reform and focused attention on the problems encountered by working class patients in obtaining health care. But this does not seem to have been so. Navarro bases his argument on insufficient evidence: quotes from George Bernard Shaw and Harold Laski and, closer to the concerns of the labour movement, a brief discussion of the annual conferences of the Labour Party from 1932 to 1934.[2] A more thorough examination of the issues debated within the Labour Party and the Trades Union Congress (TUC) — the two major representatives of the interests of the organised working class — casts doubt on his thesis.

In a general sense, the degree of radicalisation of the working class may be measured in terms of the level of strike activity (which was not high during the thirties and early forties) and the content of labour's demands.[3] But, more specifically, I take it to refer to the content and frequency of working class demands for reform within the health services. Radicalisation refers to widespread demands for comprehensive reform of the health services, rather than mere elaborations or modifications of the existing health care system. Such demands could involve a variety of proposals. At the least, they would call for the changes which the NHS achieved — a comprehensive health service free at the time of use, publicly financed, and nationally organised. Beyond this, they might call for a community based service with salaried doctors, a measure of community control in evaluation and planning, a strong emphasis on preventive as well as curative care and, more radical yet, fundamental changes in the class structure of British society, to which class differences in health can be traced.[4] They might also reject the traditional organisation and power of the medical profession, the mechanistic models of modern scientific medicine and the principles upon which the existing health services were founded — the type of rejection which we see in the post-liberation changes in China and, at the same time, in some contemporary critiques of medicine.[5] Radical demands might thus be expressed in several different plans for change, but they must represent something beyond a simple extension or modification of the existing health care system; something qualitatively different from National Health Insurance. Yet it is this — the improvement and extension of National Health Insurance — which preoccupied the Labour Party and the TUC during the twenties and thirties.

The TUC and Reform of Health Services

The response of the unions to the problems within the health services was to focus on a limited number of specific issues. Rather than addressing itself to complete reform of the health system, the union movement focused on particular issues of most immediate relevance to workers. Resolutions passed by annual TUC conferences during the twenties and thirties give little indication of the conceptualisation of a qualitatively different health system and deputations to successive Ministers of Health reflected the same concern with particular circumscribed issues as did the conference resolutions. Indeed, it is difficult to find evidence of the movement being in the forefront of pressures for reform of the health services. In the annual conferences from 1920 onwards, the health care issues uppermost in the minds of delegates reflected the problems most immediately experienced by workers — the coverage provided by National Health Insurance. Little attention was paid to problems in access to hospital care and not until the early forties was there extensive discussion of the need for a universal, comprehensive national health service. Until the early forties, the TUC saw the interests of workers as being served by more limited reforms. Let us look at these specific issues a little more closely.

Issues of Debate During the Twenties and Thirties

During the twenties and thirties, the predominant concerns of the TUC centred around the varying benefits provided by different Approved Societies; the different limits and benefits for sickness and unemployment insurance, and the inadequate coverage for dependents and for non-manual workers. Otherwise, congress resolutions were generally responses to immediate threats such as reductions in government grants to Approved Societies and reductions in benefits.

The problem of inequalities in medical benefits from different Approved Societies was never resolved but various solutions were proposed. Some delegates favoured the nationalisation of the funds of the societies while others opted for the pooling and sharing of a portion of their surpluses. At the 1925 congress, one delegate moved that:

> in view of the present unsatisfactory differing rates of benefit under the existing scheme of National Health Insurance, this Congress calls upon the Labour Movement to secure the adoption of a scheme for the nationalisation of the assets and liabilities of the whole of the Approved Societies and the equalisation of benefits payable for the equal contribution.[6]

The motion was, however, defeated and one speaker probably expressed the sentiments of many when he argued that larger surpluses (and thus more extensive benefits) were a reflection of the greater efficiency of some societies and that this efficiency might be destroyed if they were to lose their autonomy. Nationalisation was difficult to accept since it would threaten the autonomy of the unions in their capacity as Approved Societies. The importance of this role is seen in the periodic exhortations to union members to join trade union societies, rather than contributing to the growing power of the private insurance companies with whom they competed for subscribers. In 1929 for example, it was successfully moved that:

> This Congress views with concern the growing power of the great insurance corporations over National Health Insurance. To remedy this and to keep working class funds in working class organisations, it is now urged upon all workers who are members of Approved Societies run-and controlled by capitalist insurance companies that consideration should be given to the question of transferring to a Trade Union Approved Society. In addition every effort should be made to ensure that young people entering insurance for the first time should join a Trade Union Approved Society.[7]

The issue of unequal benefits was discussed again in 1932 and it was proposed that the only way in which the scheme could be truly national was for finances to be centralised and the Approved Society system to be abolished.[8] While the resolution of which this proposal formed one part was carried, dissenting delegates (from the National Federation of Insurance Workers) opposed the abolition of the societies, yet did support the principle of centralising finances through the partial pooling of surplus funds. One delegate noted that:

> The support of the insurance workers is limited so far as the centralisation of finance is concerned to the support of pooling or partial pooling of funds and the restoration of the original State grant, and does not imply the abolition of Approved Societies. We do not think it would be a benefit nor advance the objects of the resolution if the Trade Union Approved Societies or the Friendly Society Approved Societies were abolished and replaced by an administrative machine similar to that of Unemployment Insurance. One of the dangers of an unfettered bureaucratic control of National Health Insurance would be the imposition of a Means Test. So far as the payment of National Health Insurance Benefit is concerned, it must not be lost sight of that so long as you have powerful Approved Societies, so long as you have representatives of the workers responsible for the administration of them, you have a check upon bureaucratic tendency of that character.[9]

The question of divergent benefits continued to be an issue throughout the thirties and was the subject of several deputations to the Minister of Health.[10] But no governmental action was taken to cope with the problem and only with the introduction of the NHS was it resolved.

A second theme running through the annual TUC resolutions concerned the discrepancies in limits and benefits for sickness and unemployment insurance. For example, in 1930, the following successful motion was proposed by a delegate of the Insurance Workers Federation:

> This Congress urges the Government to provide rates of benefit payable for sickness and disablement within the National Health Insurance Acts equal to those payable for unemployment, and that benefits be payable for wives and dependents as under the Unemployment Insurance Acts.[11]

It was pointed out that a man over 21 years of age was entitled to 15s. per week in sickness benefit for the first 26 weeks of illness, and 7s.6d.

a week thereafter. No increases in benefit were payable for dependents. But, the same man, assuming he was married with two children, was entitled to 30s. a week in unemployment benefit. The response of Arthur Greenwood, the Labour Minister of Health, to a deputation concerned with this issue was to point out the financial obstacles to such reform; the cost of equalising benefits would amount to £8,000,000 a year, money which might be more usefully spent in improving the service. He also argued that sickness was of more transitory nature than unemployment and did not, therefore, warrant the higher level of benefits which were necessary in the case of long term unemployment.[12] As in the case of unequal benefits between different Approved Societies, no government action was taken to resolve the problem.

A third issue to which the TUC periodically directed its attention was that of the coverage for non-manual workers under National Health Insurance. For example, in the 1930 annual congress at Nottingham, it was resolved that:

> This congress requests the government to introduce, as soon as possible, legislation increasing the existing wages limit for non-manual workers in National Health and Unemployment Insurance from £250 per annum to £500 per annum, having in mind that there is no wages limit in the case of manual workers.[13]

Despite the clear specification of the new limit desired, a deputation to the Minister of Health in February 1931 said that the figure was 'more or less arbitrary' and could lie anywhere between £350 and £500 — a dubious bargaining strategy![14] In defending the increased limits the deputation noted that, amongst other things, the personal cost of obtaining medical care for men earning between £250 and £500 as non-manual workers was 'extraordinarily high'. It was argued that their inclusion would improve the panel service and that this would result in a better standard of service for all patients. But the government was reluctant to take action. In reply, the Minister argued that the medical profession was unlikely to welcome the addition of 600,000 new patients to the panel scheme, and that, quite apart from the probable opposition of doctors and employers, National Health Insurance could not absorb the additional costs of extending and increasing benefits.[15] The issue was raised again in 1934 and 1939 and the resolutions presented to the Minister, but the limit was not raised until 1941.

Such were some of the specific concerns of the union movement during the twenties and thirties. Both the content of resolutions at annual TUC conferences — few of which even related to reform of the health services — and the range of issues raised in deputations to Ministers of Health, show little interest in radical reform of the health care system. The main concern was with improving the operation of National Health Insurance and extending it to certain categories of workers, and even here, there was frequent disagreement on appropriate solutions as each union sought to protect its own interests.

Pressures for a State Medical Service

It was not until the early forties that the TUC seriously considered more radical reform of the health system. This interest was partly a response to government initiatives; not until the establishment of the Interdepartmental Committee on Social Insurance and Allied Services, headed by Beveridge, did the TUC consider the establishment of a comprehensive and universal national health service. One resolution at the 1920 conference had envisaged a considerable reorganisation of the health system and proposed that

> a full and efficient medical service be instituted and the provision of clinics, dispensaries, hospitals, doctors and nurses throughout the kingdom under the Ministry of Health. That all the present hospitals, dispensaries, Poor Law infirmaries and institutions be taken over for the purpose and the moneys necessary be provided by Parliament and local authorities.[16]

Yet the issue was not pursued in the years which followed.

Insofar as general reforms were debated during the inter-war years, they were of a less comprehensive nature. For example, the 1930 congress voiced a concern with the nature of the medical care which was available to workers. Emphasis was placed on the wide gap between the state of medical knowledge and the actual practice of medicine and it was noted this gap was particularly marked in the care of working class patients: 'The wife of the average workman does not get the same attention as was displayed at Glamis Castle a few days ago.'[17] Another delegate dwelt on the priority which doctors gave to private rather than panel patients.[18] It was moved by the congress that

> This congress directs the General Council to approach the Government with a view to consultation taking place between the Government, the British Medical Association and the General Council, for the purpose of considering the steps that should be taken to secure

more adequate services for the money expended, especially having regard to the fact that the application of known medical science by the practitioner is a very long way behind the discoveries made.[19]

In the discussion of the resolution and also in the report of the deputation to the Minister of Health, it is clear that the unions were concerned with providing specialist care to workers and both general and specialist care to their dependents. But these concerns did not lead to proposals for a comprehensive reorganisation of the health care sector. Ernest Bevin was envisaging the development of 'co-operative' medicine:

> Supposing you had in a working class district, instead of a number of badly built surgeries with people standing in queues and getting worse colds than the one they came to have cured —supposing you could get a dozen or twenty doctors equipped with proper clinics, able to co-operate and able to contribute to each other's knowledge with the opportunity and time to specialise in diagnosis, when new diseases arise we should not have to wait for years for them to be discovered, but right out on the circumference where the actual working man and woman is being treated we should be gathering knowledge in order to grapple with the disease more readily than we can at the present moment.[20]

Considerable emphasis was placed on a co-operative approach to the problem of providing good health care and it was envisaged that the government, the medical profession and the unions could together address themselves to the problem. Bevin asked the congress to approach this problem 'not in the scramble of a political struggle, but on a basis of consideration and investigation'.[21]

It is interesting to note that the professional organisation with which co-operation was sought was the BMA and not the Socialist Medical Association (SMA), which claimed to represent the interests of workers and which had already drawn the outline of a medical service based on socialist principles.[22] Seven years later the BMA and the TUC formed a joint committee concerned with 'general health questions, and, in particular, research and the training of doctors in industrial diseases, as well as other matters, such as National Health Insurance and factory legislation'.[23] One delegate at the 1937 congress moved that there should also be co-operation with the SMA and noted that this body had affiliated with the Labour Party and was helping to formulate its health policy. He argued that the BMA was bitterly opposed to the proposals of the SMA and pointed out that the BMA was representative of the 'individualistic and unprogressive' outlook of the bulk of the medical profession'.[24] Yet no delegate was willing to second the motion and allow a discussion of the issue. The TUC showed little willingness to align itself with those who claimed to be working towards a national health service founded on socialist principles. It is not clear why this was so, unless the TUC chose, for pragmatic reasons, to align itself with the more powerful representative of the medical profession.

The issues raised in 1930 were returned to again in 1932. This time the congress more explicitly stated its concern with centralising the finances of National Health Insurance, abolishing the panel system and establishing a state medical service which would provide services for the dependents of workers and which would include specialist, maternity, dental and optical services.[25] Yet there was still no consideration of a universal and comprehensive state medical service. It was not until 1940 that the TUC returned to a more general consideration of reform of health services. Dr L.W. Hefferman of the Medical Practitioners' Union moved that

> in view of the waste of effort and money in connection with the existing Medical Services by reason of overlapping, duplication and lack of co-ordination, and in particular the failure to provide a home medical service for large sections of the community who are unable to provide it for themselves, and having regard to the vital necessity of maintaining the health of the nation, this congress presses upon the Government the importance of instituting at the earliest possible moment, and preliminary to a National Medical Service, a General Practitioner Service free to all.[26]

The motion envisaged the eventual introduction of a more comprehensive service, and, believing 'Germany's defeat is merely a matter of time and material', Hefferman advocated that the first step towards such a service be taken as soon as possible. The matter was remitted to the General Council for consideration. It is interesting to note that it was a representative of the medical profession who urged the Council to 'take more note of these medical matters, because the subject is of supreme importance to the workers and their families. These people look to the Trade Union movement and their executive personnel, not only to take heed but to implement the decisions of Congress'.[27] Indeed, the TUC appears to have been rather slow in evolving a policy concerning reform of the health services. Various groups within the medical profession had by this time developed quite detailed plans for the reorganisation of health services, yet the union movement still lacked a clear policy. This emerges in the comments of one delegate who spoke to the 1940 resolution:

> I am very doubtful, and I hope that Congress will be doubtful, that this is the moment that we should pass a Resolution saying that a general practitioner service free to all should necessarily form the basis of our future National Medical Service. If we are working towards a National Medical Service we have to watch very carefully each step that we are to take. We have the whole position of the Local Authorities' Medical Services to consider. I believe that the General Council, in discussing this matter, have been trying to work out a scheme whereby the two should be co-ordinated, and I feel very strongly that it is very doubtful whether a free general practitioner service based entirely on the general practitioner is the first preliminary step to a National Medical Service, in view of all the Local Authority development of health services.[28]

It was in 1940 that the General Council of the TUC concluded that a complete reform of National Health Insurance and related social services was necessary.[29] Early in 1941 the Minister of Health received a deputation from the General Council. They drew to the Minister's attention the content of Congress resolutions of previous years: variations in benefits between Approved Societies; differences in income limits and benefits between Health Insurance and Unemployment Insurance; the inadequate provision of medical benefits; and the failure of National Health Insurance to provide proper records for research purposes. In the light of such problems 'The Minister was urged to make a comprehensive examination of the whole position with a view to getting a worthwhile Scheme under way'.[30] The response to the delegation's concerns was more positive than had previously been the case — quite apart from announcing proposed increases in health insurance benefits and in the income limit for non-manual workers, the Minister noted that the government had been addressing itself to these matters before the 'blitz' and that it was initiating a comprehensive review of all social insurance schemes in order to prepare for post-war reforms.[31] In effect, the TUC was entering the debate over reform at a relatively late stage and its General Council was compelled to more fully develop plans for reform in order to present evidence to the Inter-departmental Committee on Social Insurance and Allied Services, headed by Sir William Beveridge.

The General Council submitted a memorandum to the committee and also appeared before it on two occasions in 1942. The bulk of the submission was concerned with levels of benefits, eligibility and contributions. Their stance on the reform of health services was summarised as follows:

> A comprehensive national medical service covering everything that medical science can command for prevention and cure of sickness should be provided by the nation and made available to everybody in the State. This service should include a statistical department for the provision of occupational and geographical records necessary to safeguard the health of the people. There should also be associated with the medical services a complete rehabilitation service on up-to-date lines.[32]

They foresaw the abolition of Approved Societies and argued that local authorities should be responsible for administering services. They did, however, envisage a continued though unclear role for bodies such as trade unions which, 'with their long and honourable tradition of service ought to be preserved so that the benefit of their experience and good will can be utilised in administration on behalf of the State'.[33] This was the first time that the union movement committed itself to a universal and comprehensive state medical service. But far from being in the forefront of pressures for reform, it lagged behind the medical profession in evolving plans for reform and pressuring for change. Despite the fact that one branch of the medical profession — the SMA — was pressuring for a socialist medical service, the TUC did not choose to align itself with this body. The sense we have is of a movement whch responded to events rather than itself initiating action.

Labour Party Policy

A review of the reports of annual conferences of the Labour Party from 1920, indicates a concern with the same specific issues as the TUC. Early publications, largely the work of the party's Public Health Advisory Committee, which received considerable input from members of the medical profession, do not appear to have shaped the discussion of reform at conferences during the twenties.[34] Apart from these and a conference on 'The Hospital Problem' organised in 1924 by the Executive Committee of the party and bringing together groups representing labour, hospitals and the medical profession, there was little attention

devoted to broader issues of reform until the early thirties.[35] Even
then, discussions took place largely at the prompting of a medical
pressure group — the SMA. Dr Somerville Hastings of the SMA spoke
on behalf of the Labour Party at the 1924 conference and it was he
who successfully introduced resolutions on the planning of a state
medical service. Between 1930 and 1933, district branches of the party
submitted a total of fourteen resolutions asking for comprehensive
reform of health services — obviously, there was at this time some
interest in comprehensive reform among the membership of the party
— but only the SMA resolution appears in the reports of the annual
conferences.[36] It was in 1932 that Hastings (seconded by another
doctor) successfully moved:

> That in the opinion of this conference the health needs of the
> country can only be effectively provided by the establishment of a
> complete State Medical Service, giving everything necessary for the
> prevention and treatment of disease, free and open to all; and that
> the National Executive Committee be requested to report upon the
> subject, particularly in its relations to the Social Services generally.[37]

But though the resolution was carried, the acceptance of SMA policy
by the Labour Party was slow to cystallise. At the 1924 conference,
the secretary of the party's Public Health Advisory Committee had said
that all the party asked for was efficiency,[38] and the same caution
can be detected in the chairman's comments following Hasting's resolution — 'I must not be understood as offering any objection to this resolution, but I should be failing in my duty if I did not point out that the
implications of it, desirable as they may be — and I do not deny it — are
very far-reaching'.[39] Because it 'had to deal with a fairly wide range of
important and complicated subjects',[40] the National Executive delayed
consideration of the resolution until 1934, and even then it issued a
rather brief and cautious preliminary report.[41]

It was not until 1943 that the Labour Party accepted SMA policy.
Recognising a wide range of problems within the health sector, the
party's first major statement of policy on health services, *National
Service for Health*, called for the organisation of a universal, comprehensive national health service under the Ministry of Health, with the
responsibility for organising health centres and hospital services lying in
the hands of democratically elected regional health authorities.[42] The
service would be financed through taxation and rates, it would be free at
the time of use and the medical profession was to be employed on a full

time salaried basis. The ultimate goal was a unified hospital system but at first, voluntary hospitals would receive payment for cases referred to them, with local authorities receiving commensurate representation on their governing boards. It was anticipated that, before long, the effect of such a policy would be to bring the voluntary hospitals under the control of local authorities. Preventive care was emphasised and it was recognised that the goal of improved health would only be achieved by broader social and economic changes, though the way in which these changes were conceptualised represented no explicit challenge to class relations in British society:

> We need social action to create the conditions under which the healthy needs of the whole population can be satisfied. In truth, there is hardly any activity of government which does not affect health directly or indirectly. If, through a sound social and economic policy, we can master poverty, we shall thereby do much to eliminate ill-health; for poverty is still the greatest single cause of ill-health. If, by good government, we secure for all good conditions of work, with full employment, and with ample opportunity for leisure and exercise; if, through our public services, the citizen can obtain well-built and well-placed houses, with sanitation, water, clean and plentiful milk and other nourishing food, clean air and as much sunlight as possible, and freedom from injurious noise; then the health of the nation will benefit far more from these causes than from much doctoring.[43]

But the party was slow in reaching this point and played little part in shaping or creating a public debate over reform of the health services. It is difficult to construe this history of concern with health care as representing a pressing demand for radical reform. Though there was dissatisfaction with National Health Insurance, this remained at the level of specific issues, and the idea of a state medical service was developed largely at the prompting of members of the medical profession, most particularly the SMA. Even these pressures only reached fruition after the debate over reform had already been placed in the public arena by the publication of the Beveridge Report.[44] As in the case of the TUC, the image is of a party responding to, rather than creating events.

Conclusion

There is little evidence of the radicalisation of the working class; the concerns of organised labour focused largely on the improvement and extension of National Health Insurance; the Labour Party was slow to respond to the pressures of the SMA and the TUC chose to collaborate with the BMA. In the light of the broad range of problems which existed within the health services and given the nature of these working class concerns with reform, we cannot explain the NHS simply as a response to the demands of the working class. The policy of the TUC and the Labour Party did become more well defined and more radical by the early forties, but at this point they were entering rather than initiating a public debate. We may also note that even these more radical conceptions of change were hardly a threatening socialist alternative; they represented no real threat to capital and posed no challenge to the power of the medical profession. Indeed, members of the profession had helped shape the policy and a significant proportion of the profession was in accord with the proposals.

Notes

1. Vicente Navarro, *Class Struggle, The State and Medicine* (Martin Robertson, London, 1978). For a similar thesis with respect to the growth of social welfare legislation in general see R. Miliband, *The State in Capitalist Society* (Quartet, London, 1969), p. 99; J. Strachey, *Contemporary Capitalism* (Victor Gollancz, London, 1956), p. 154; Dorthy Wedderburn (ed.), *Poverty, Inequality and Class Structure* (Cambridge University Press, London, 1974), pp. 142-3.
2. Navarro, *Class Struggle*, pp. 26-9.
3. For data on strike activity see George Sayer Bain, Robert Bacon and John Pimlott, 'The Labour Force' in A.H. Halsey (ed.), *Trends in British Society Since 1900: A Guide to the Changing Social Structure of Britain* (Macmillan, London,, 1972), Table 4.14. Runciman argues that during the interwar years 'the most obvious comparative reference group for the prosperous manual worker was still other workers less fortunate than himself'. These other workers experienced severe hardships, but militant discontent was never widespread and the majority of the victims of the Depression appear to have thought of themselves as 'victims of misfortune rather than injustice'. The relative absence of social and political protest may be intelligible in terms of the low level of deprivation felt by workers because of limited reference groups. W.G. Runciman, *Relative Deprivation and Social Justice* (Routledge and Kegan Paul, London, 1966), pp. 57-77.
4. Class differences in health are discussed in Ch. 7.
5. Analyses of changes in the Chinese health-care system can be found in J.S. Horn, *Away With All Pests* (Bantam, New York, 1972); Matthew H. Liang, Philip S. Eichling, Lawrence J. Fine and George J. Annas, 'Chinese Health Care: Determinants of the System', *American Journal of Public Health*, vol. 63, no. 2 (February 1973), pp. 102-10; S.B. Rifkin, 'Public Health in China – Is the Experience Relevant to Other Less Developed Nations?', *Social Science and Medicine*, vol. 7 (1973), pp. 249-57; V.W. Sidel, 'Some Observations on the Health Services in the People's Republic of China', *International Journal of Health Services*, vol. 2, no. 3 (1972), pp. 385-95. Among the contemporary critiques of

medicine are Hans Peter Dreitzel (ed.), *The Social Organization of Health* (Macmillan, New Yo.ʳ, 1971), pp. v-xvii; Marc Renaud, 'On the Structural Constraints to State Intervention in Health', *International Journal of Health Services*, vol. 5, no. 4 (1975), pp. 559-71; Martin Rossdale, 'Health in a Sick Society', *New Left Review*, vol. 34 (1965), pp. 82-91.

6. The Trades Union Congress, *Report of the Proceedings of the 57th Annual Trades Union Congress* (The Trades Union Congress, London, 1925), p. 525.

7. Ibid., *Report of the Proceedings of the 61st Annual Trades Union Congress* (1929), p. 372.

8. Ibid., *Report of the Proceedings of the 64th Annual Trades Union Congress* (1932), pp. 286-7.

9. Ibid., p. 288.

10. Ibid., *Report of the Proceedings of the 70th Annual Trades Union Congress* (1938), p. 335; *Report of the Proceedings of the 73rd Annual Trades Union Congress* (1941), p. 238.

11. Ibid., *Report of the Proceedings of the 62nd Annual Trades Union Congress* (1930), p. 320.

12. Ibid., *Report of the Proceedings of the 63rd Annual Trades Union Congress* (1931), p. 154.

13. Ibid., *62nd Congress*, p. 293.

14. Ibid., *63rd Congress*, p. 152.

15. Ibid., p. 154.

16. Ibid., *Report of the Proceedings of the 52nd Annual Trades Union Congress* (1920), p. 362.

17. Ibid., *62nd Congress*, p. 321.

18. Ibid., p. 322.

19. Ibid., p. 321.

20. Ibid., p. 322.

21. Ibid.

22. The proposals of the BMA and the SMA are discussed in Ch. 5. Both were in favour of some form of state medical service but the proposals of the SMA were somewhat more radical.

23. The Trades Union Congress, *Report of the Proceedings of the 69th Annual Trades Union Congress* (1938), p. 130.

24. Ibid., p. 343.

25. Ibid., *64th Congress*, pp. 286-9.

26. Ibid., *Report of the Proceedings of the 72nd Annual Trades Union Congress* (1940), p. 349.

27. Ibid., p. 350.

28. Ibid.

29. Ibid., *73rd Congress*, p. 114.

30. Ibid.

31. Ibid.

32. Ibid., *Report of the Proceedings of the 74th Annual Trades Union Congress* (1942) p. 40.

33. Ibid.

34. The Labour Party, Memoranda Prepared by the Advisory Committee on Public Health. I. *The Organisation of the Preventative and Curative Medical Services and Hospital and Laboratory Systems Under a Ministry of Health* (The Labour Party, London, 1919); The Trades Union Congress and The Labour Party, *The Labour Movement and the Hospital Crisis: A Statement of Policy With Regard to Hospitals* (The Trades Union Congress and the Labour Party, London, 1922); Ibid., *The Labour Movement and Preventive and Curative Medical Services: A Statement of Policy With Regard to Health.* (The Trades Union Congress and the Labour Party, London, 1923). The first of these laid the basis for the subsequent

publications and it is discussed in Ch. 5. I have taken it to represent the views of certain members of the medical profession because over half of the committee membership was drawn from the profession and because the proposals contained in these reports were not the basis of discussions of reform within the TUC; they were not used by congress delegates to formulate plans for reform and to press for change.

35. The Labour Party, *The Hospital Problem* (The Labour Party, London, 1924).

36. Ibid., *Agenda for the 30th Annual Conference* (The Labour Party, London, 1930); Ibid., *Agenda for the 31st Annual Conference* (1931); Ibid., *Agenda for the 32nd Annual Conference* (1932).

37. Ibid., *Report of the 32nd Annual Conference* (The Labour Party, London, 1932), p. 269.

38. Ibid., *The Hospital Problem*.

39. Ibid., *Report of the 32nd Conference*, p. 270.

40. Ibid., *Report of the 33rd Annual Conference* (1933), p. 141.

41. Ibid., *Report of the 34th Annual Conference* (1934), pp. 256-8.

42. Ibid., *National Service for Health* (The Labour Party, London, 1943).

43. Ibid., p.2.

44. Sir William Beveridge, *Report on Social Insurance and Allied Services* (HMSO, London, 1942).

5 THE MEDICAL PROFESSION AND REFORM OF THE HEALTH SERVICES

It is most frequently assumed that the extensive provision of public medical services is contrary to the interests of the medical profession, and the introduction of varying forms of socialised medicine has been taken as evidence of the state acting in the interests of patients — particularly working class patients — and against those of the medical profession.[1] Many writers would agree with Navarro's observation that 'most of the changes in . . . health services have occurred not because but in spite of the medical profession'.[2] This image of conflict between the profession and the state is based upon and reinforced by the fact that where public medical care programmes have been introduced, there has been vocal opposition from the medical profession, often culminating in strikes or the threat of such.[3]

This opposition of the profession to any form of socialised medicine, while seldom explained in detail, is seen to flow from the threat to professional autonomy which the state poses. State intervention is viewed as depriving the profession of control over the setting and actual practice of medicine, for it threatens third party intervention in the doctor-patient relationship, and freedom and initiative are endangered by the bureaucratisation which is considered to be an undoubted corollary of state involvement.[4] Implicit within such perceptions of conflict is an image of a profession which is autonomous, which does have considerable freedom to determine conditions of practice, and which has developed as a community of laissez-faire medical entrepreneurs, relatively unconstrained by either state or consumer. Socialised medicine is seen to represent the antithesis of this tradition of professional autonomy.

But these images of the profession's response to state intervention in the health sector appear to be overly simplistic and they fail to adequately account for the fact that, at times, an extension of the state's function in providing health care has been encouraged by the profession. From the 1920s until the early forties the medical profession in Britain was proposing the extension of state medical services and did not see this as necessarily opposed to its interests. The profession appears to have played an active part in defining problems within the health sector and shaping the debate over the form which a new service should assume. This in itself is not remarkable, for we would expect that those working within the health sector would be concerned with safeguarding and pursuing their interests by seeking to direct the course of change. What is remarkable, given common assumptions, is the fact that the medical profession was proposing a considerable extension of the state's function in providing health care. Without exception, the various branches of the profession which issued reports during the inter-war years, were in favour of some more or less extensive state medical service. Also, it is important to note that in these various proposals for change, the major emphasis was on rationalising the organisation and financing of medical services. While class inequalities in access to health care were recognised, these were seen as one of several different types of problems. Once again, there is little evidence to support the thesis that the NHS was largely a response to class conflict and to the poor access of working class patients to care.

This is not to argue that some form of socialised medicine was un-animously favoured within the profession: it was not. At times the wis-dom of proposals for an extension of public medical services was hotly disputed. Some physicians were vehemently opposed to such plans and saw them in the nature of a 'totalitarian nightmare', while others were clearly ambivalent and though they felt that the state must assume responsibility for planning a unified national health service with publicly financed medical care available for the bulk of the population, they were also mindful of the threat to professional freedoms which this might entail. Yet these doubts only helped to justify the active debate over reform and the energies invested in formulating proposals for change, for only in this way could the profession hope to prevent any scheme being foisted upon it. Friedson distinguishes two aspects of professional control — over the social aspects of practice and over the social and economic organisation of work.[5] The former — autonomy of technique — he sees as the distinguishing characteristic of a profession. The latter varies as relationships between profession and state vary, but 'lack of control over the socio-economic terms of work do not signifi-cantly change its essential character as a profession'.[6] The majority of the medical profession in Britain did not appear to view further state intervention in the health sector as necessarily threatening their autonomy of technique and insofar as the social organisation of their work would be more open to external controls, this was not viewed as ultimately being contrary to the interests of the profession.

This is not altogether surprising if, instead of assuming professional autonomy, we recognise that the bulk of the medical profession in Britain had enjoyed a limited freedom in determining the social organisation of their work. If we recognise that the autonomy which some physicians wished to preserve was something of an illusion, then the profession's proposals for a national health service become intelligible. For many decades, the majority of physicians had worked in some form of contract practice or institutional context which had the effect of limiting their autonomy. Even in the latter part of the nineteenth century, the individual practitioner catering solely to private patients was an anomaly. Many doctors worked in contract with employers, friendly societies, medical missions, trade unions, National Health Insurance, the Poor Law or local authorities. While the ideology of the profession emphasised the freedom of the individual practitioner to create his own conditions of work and of patients to freely choose their physicians, such freedoms were limited. No doubt this tradition of control of physicians made the idea of a public medical service less threatening and less fraught with imaginary dangers. Moreover, the majority of doctors had financially benefited from the introduction of National Health Insurance and even in 1917, the British Medical Association (BMA) was willing to contemplate its extension.[7]

Thus the acceptance of an extension of public medical services is intelligible in terms of the profession's past experience; physicians had already relinquished a large measure of control over the social organisation of their work, a tradition of consumer control was already established, and practice within the public medical sector had proved to be lucrative while not limiting basic professional freedoms. But the willingness to contemplate an extension of public medical services was not only manifested during the inter-war years; the profession had, in fact, exhibited such a willingness in earlier decades. Titmuss notes that the *British Medical Journal* was suggesting state assistance in obtaining health care for workers before Lloyd George's proposals for National Health Insurance were known.[8] And Hodgkinson argues that 'in the breakdown of laissez-faire principles the whole medical profession in the nineteenth century played a dominant part';[9] as one of the new groups of experts, they were 'the first scientific individualists to co-operate with state collectivism':[10]

> Had it not been for the pressure of the first public doctors, sometimes individually but generally collectively through their associations, it is doubtful whether many of the developments would have come in the country's medical system . . . It is these doctors, now all forgotten and unrecognised, who were the fathers of the twentieth century State Medical Service.[11]

The profession had by no means totally opposed an extension of the functions of the state in providing health care. Insofar as there was vehement opposition to Lloyd George's proposals for National Health Insurance, this was directed against the particular conditions under which they were asked to join the plan and the levels of remuneration; there was little opposition to the principle of the scheme. As Brand indicates, 'The manner in which the Act had been framed, with almost no consultation with representatives of the medical profession, had been responsible for much of the uproar.'[12]

This involvement in the process of reform and the profession's acceptance of the state's increasing responsibility in the provision of health care continued throughout the twenties, thirties and early forties. During these decades, a steady stream of reports was issued by bodies representing various branches of the medical profession. These in turn helped to promote considerable debate over the need for reform and the most appropriate manner of reorganising the health services. In these reports, as in the correspondence columns, lead articles and addresses appearing in the *British Medical Journal* and *Lancet*, we see the health services being critically evaluated and schemes for reorganisation being advanced. Without exception, these reports recommended an extension of the state's function in the health care sector.

Identification of Problems Within the Health Services

Of the several publications issued during the inter-war years, in which different sections of the medical profession sought to identify the most obvious deficiencies of the health services and advance proposals for reform, our starting point is the 1919 memorandum of the Labour Party's Advisory Committee on Public Health. I include this here because over half the committee membership was drawn from the medical profession.[13] This was followed in 1920 by the Dawson Report, an interim report prepared for the Minister of Health by the Consultative Council on Medical and Allied Services, which drew its membership from the elite of the medical professon.[14] The BMA issued several publications during this period, the major statements of its cautious policy being the reports of 1929 and 1938.[15] More radical in conception were the proposals of the Socialist Medical Association (SMA) published in 1933[16] and the plans for reorganisation of the hospital services put forward by the 'Special Commissioner' of *Lancet* in 1939.[17] There followed in 1942 the Draft Interim Report of the Medical Planning Commission[18] — which had been organised by the BMA and the Royal Colleges — and the interim statement of policy of

Medical Planning Research, a more radical body which had been established to represent the views of the younger members of the profession.[19]

These reports prompted addresses and lead articles on the issue of reform, and provoked debates in the correspondence columns of the British Medical Journal and Lancet — most particularly from 1938 onwards. Members of the BMA were urged to establish local groups to discuss the various proposals for reform and to facilitate such discussion, the British Medical Journal published a series of short yet comprehensive reviews of the issues which had been raised.[20] Each of these sources gives us an indication of the profession's definitions of the problems within the health services and also demonstrates the general readiness to advocate some form of public medical service.

A continuing theme in these various sources was the need to rationalise the organisation of health services — to unify and co-ordinate services and to make more efficient use of resources. Relatively little attention was devoted to issues of class inequality. The 1919 memorandum of the Labour Party's Advisory Committee on Public Health noted the health problems of the working class: 'In Finsbury the death rate per 1,000 of infants has been found to vary from 41 in well-to-do districts to 375 in the slums.'[21] It saw this as a social rather than a medical problem — preventive medicine may help to reduce these inequalities, but ultimately the problem lies in differences in 'industrial and housing conditions, due largely to exploitation of land, which have led to the most serious deterioration of national health and happiness'.[22] Yet it was recognised that low income patients were often the first beneficiaries of scientific medicine: 'the poor who go to a hospital with a medical school often secure a more accurate diagnosis and treatment than the patients of a private doctor'.[23] In the case of wealthier patients, time is spent on practising the 'art of medicine' — visiting, humouring and encouraging patients — rather than the 'science of medicine'. But if anything, the most disadvantaged section of the population was neither the rich nor the poor but 'the men and women who are neither one nor the other'. Ineligible for free or subsidised care, they could not afford the increasing costs of private medical care, and while 'the importance of institutional treatment is becoming more and more recognised . . . under present conditions most of the middle classes are excluded from its benefits. They cannot afford nursing homes, and they are not eligible for the voluntary hospitals'.[24]

The problems of middle income families were also recognised by others. In 1942 the British Medical Journal noted that 'A full institutional service . . . is more easily available to the rich and to the poor than to the middle classes'.[25] In its interim policy statement, Medical Planning Research argued that the 'middle classes can obtain the same admirable service available to the rich — but only at a price which adds financial to physical distress'.[26] Yet it did not see the rich as being free from problems, for while they could pay for high quality care, they were 'in grave danger of falling into the hands of pseudo-consultants, medical rogues, charlatans and tricksters, who exploit the Harley Street neighbourhood in the absence of any publicly recognisable guarantee of consultant efficiency'.[27] In no report was the main emphasis placed upon the problems that working class patients experienced in obtaining medical care. For at least one physician on whose comments *Lancet* reported, such an emphasis would have been entirely inappropriate: 'Possibly, we . . . [are] pampering the public too much financially; the working class, for example, [can] afford wireless sets and visits to the cinema but they . . . [have] the idea that they ought not to pay for doctoring'.[28]

Despite the comments cited, none of the reports, articles and correspondence placed major emphasis on class inequalities in access to health care — whether it was the problems of the working class or of the middle class. Instead, the focus was on a range of organisational issues; problems arising from the financial base of the hospitals; the poor co-ordination between the numerous units responsible for providing care; the maldistribution of services and facilities; the isolation of the general practitioner; the burden of the initial capital outlay in setting up practice; and the doubtful viability of private consulting practice. While these organisational problems were related to problems of class inequality, these links were seldom emphasised.

In 1920, the Dawson Report drew attention to the problems of the voluntary hospitals:

That the hospitals have fallen on evil days is known to all. The reason is two-fold. One is that the prices of all the commodities a hospital has to buy — its coal, food, linen, etc. as well as the salaries and wages it has to pay, have increased. The other reason is that the investigation and treatment of disease are becoming increasingly complex. So that not only are the old items of expenditure more costly, but there is hardly a year but some new method of diagnosis or treatment makes it necessary to incur fresh expenditure, and capital expenditure in a hospital differs from capital expenditure in business, in that when a business house grows, it grows in earning capacity. And therefore, almost without exception every hospital in the country is facing increasing difficulty in carrying on its work.[29]

The Labour Party's Advisory Committee on Public Health had also noted the financial difficulties of the voluntary hospitals and claimed that 'some of the present hospitals are not as efficiently equipped as they should be' and that the number of beds which were available was 'nothing like the number required'.[30] It was not only the problems of voluntary hospitals which were recognised: the 'Special Commissioner' appointed by *Lancet* pointed out that as a result of their different tax bases, 'rich counties like Middlesex and Surrey have developed a fine municipal hospital service while poor counties have all too often had to be content with public-assistance institutions'.[31]

The main focus in the 1938 statement of BMA policy is on the poorly organised and co-ordinated state of the health services which are 'different in their origin and inspiration, diverse in their form and bewildering in their complexity'.[32] They noted that the growth of the services had been largely haphazard with 'much overlapping and unnecessary complication and confusion'.[33] Though the state had been assuming an increasing responsibility in the provision of health care, this had failed to unify the health services to an appreciable extent:

It cannot be said that each new development is an expression of a unified health policy of ordered development — the result has been piecemeal and fragmentary growth rather than consistent and systematic development. The public is often served by unrelated and competitive agencies. The individual passes from local authority to voluntary body, from consulting room to clinic, or hospital, from private to official doctor and often back again, to obtain from many unrelated agencies a service which could be more efficiently provided as one co-ordinated whole. Some services are available to one citizen but not to another in similar circumstances; some serve the citizen at home, while others are prohibited from so doing; some services he obtains at public expense, others he must pay for privately.[34]

Such inconsistencies in the provision of services are not surprising, for even if we ignore the multitude of different agencies responsible for providing health care, state responsibilities alone were divided among many different branches of government; in the early forties, responsibility was shared by the Ministry of Health, the Board of Education, the Home Office, the Ministry of Pensions, the Ministry of Labour, the General Post Office, and the Ministry of Supply.[35]

Perhaps the most urgent need for planning was seen to be in the hospital system, for the attempts to achieve a measure of co-ordination during the twenties and thirties were singularly unsuccessful. The BMA remarked upon the 'Lack or insufficiency of co-operation' and the maldistribution of hospital services and the 'Special Commissioner' of *Lancet* pointed out that 'It has long been realised that England stands in need of some hospital organisation with regional planning'. He was of the opinion that, by means of the wartime Emergency Hospital Service 'Hitler and the Ministry between them accomplished in a few months what might have taken the British Hospitals' Association twenty years to bring about'.[36] Medical Planning Research also drew attention to inequalities in the services, conditions and facilities which were offered to patients:

> At one end of the scale are the best voluntary and municipal general hospitals; at the other are certain remote provincial voluntary hospitals, cottage hospitals, nursing homes and municipal fever hospitals, in which one would not wish one's worse enemies to be patients.[37]

Certain issues were more intimately linked with physicians' interests. Several reports devoted attention to the isolation and low status of the general practitioner and to the high capital costs faced by young doctors establishing themselves in a practice. The SMA noted the problems which GPs had identified:

> The chief of these disadvantages are: personal — uncertainty and variability of income, long and irregular hours, considerable capital outlay, no pension, difficulty of finding time for research and postgraduate study; professional — lack of complete facilities for all his patients, exclusion from the hospitals and clinics, inability to follow up his cases when admitted to hospital, and lack of guidance on new therapeutic methods.[38]

Some physicians saw these problems as both symbolising and accelerating the demise of the GP, and some were doubtful of the viability of private general and consulting practice during the post-war period. But the tone of most reports is less pessimistic. The Medical Planning Commission's proposals were aimed in part at reducing the sense of isolation experienced by general practitioners, which it saw as emanating from the conditions of solo practice — the exclusion of GPs from hospitals, their lack of easy access to diagnostic facilities, and limited opportunities for easy collaboration with consultants and other GPs.[39] The *British Medical Journal*, reviewing the defects of the health system from the point of view of the practitioner, emphasised the lack of recognition of the place of the GP, the unwillingness of hospital authorities to invite their co-operation, the limited opportunities for team work and for following up patients who were referred to other agencies, and the increasingly heavy burden of the large capital outlay involved in establishing a practice.[40] But few openly admitted the fears of one speaker at the 1939 Scientific Meetings of the BMA who argued that 'The general practitioner if he were wise would press for a state medical service as quickly as possible before encroachment wiped him out altogether.'[41] Though *Lancet* did note that at the BMA meetings in Aberdeen in the same year, many divisions submitted resolutions which urged the expansion of public medical services as, among other things, a means of 'maintaining the position of the general practitioner'.[42] Some physicians also predicted the decline of private consulting practice and the 'Special Commissioner' of *Lancet* based his proposals for a reorganised hospital service partly on his belief that there was unlikely to be a sufficiently high demand for private care from consultants after the war.[43]

Such were the major problems identified by the profession. The emphasis was on the many organisational and financial inadequacies of the health services and the way in which these threatened the interests of patients and physicians. But insofar as patients' interests were discussed, these were defined by the profession in accordance with its perceptions of illness and the role of medicine. Few questions were raised about the efficacy of medicine, the hierarchical organisation within the health professions and the ways in which people's needs for care might be defined. Even though the goal of improved health was often espoused in the introductions to the reports, there was little attempt to explore the bases of illness, other than in terms of traditional medical models. What this means is that the specific interests of the profession informed the definition of organisational problems. This bias is also apparent in the proposals for reform which were advanced.

Proposals for Reform

A broad area of consensus can be identified in the proposals for change which were formulated by the profession. There was general agreement that a reorganised health service would be centred around general practitioners; that the isolation of GPs would be counteracted by the introduction of health centres; that patients should have free choice of doctor; that hospital services should be organised on a regional basis; that the health services should be concerned with both preventive and curative care; and that financial considerations should prevent no one from obtaining necessary care. Even though there were variations in details, there was a consensus that the state should assume a significantly greater responsibility in the provision of medical care. At the very least, it was envisaged that National Health Insurance should be extended to the dependents of workers already covered by the scheme — thus providing coverage for about 90 per cent of the population. With the exception of some diehards, physicians debated the nature and extent of the state's function in providing health care, rather than whether such a state function was appropriate. The more heated and emotional debates were provoked by the advocates of a full time salaried service, but opposition to such proposals cannot be construed as opposition to the idea of socialised medicine *per se*. There is little support for the images of the medical profession which Foote develops in his biography of Aneurin Bevan. Foote's claim that the profession held a 'deeply entrenched belief that almost any system of state control over medicine would destroy the doctor's clinical freedom'[44] seems completely unfounded, and there is little evidence that 'Much the strongest bent in the medical mind was a non-political conservatism, a revulsion against all change, a habit of intellectual isolation which enabled them (*sic*) to magnify any proposals for reform into a totalitarian nightmare'.[45]

The main areas of dispute concerned such issues as the unification of the hospital system; methods of remunerating the profession; the proportion of the population which would be entitled to publicly financed care and the means of financing the services. It is on the basis of their position on these issues that we might label reports as radical or conservative.

Conservative Proposals

Most conservative of the proposals were those issued by the BMA during the 1930s. 'While recognising existing conditions and circumstances', it sought to 'adjust, modify and extend present services'.[46] Its aim was to produce a 'co-ordinated and, as far as possible, unified system, effective and reasonably complete', and this was to be based on four principles: that care should be both preventive and curative; that patients should receive primary care from a GP of their own choice; that consultations with specialists should only be through referrals from GPs; and that there should be co-ordination of the various services. Translated into relatively cautious proposals, these principles involved the publicly controlled reorganisation of the health services. The BMA recommended the extension of National Health Insurance coverage to the dependents of insured workers and also an extension of medical benefits such that these would include dental, ophthalmic and a full range of specialist services. Despite the fact that the Association proposed relatively few changes, it is important that we recognise that it was recommending a complete public medical service, financed through worker and employer contributions, for about 90 per cent of the population. This can hardly be labelled as opposition to socialised medicine.

That the policy of the BMA became less cautious during the 1940s is evident in the Association's response to the Draft Interim Report of the Medical Planning Commission. At the conference of BMA representatives in September 1942, the main items of debate concerned the report of the Commission. In these debates the representatives voted in favour of a comprehensive medical service for all people to be financed through contributory or insurance schemes.[47] While a motion proposing a whole-time salaried service was lost by 177 votes to 20, 'many of the speeches favoured the motion'.[48] The report of the Medical Planning Commission which had prompted such debates had been published in June of the same year.[49] The Commission drew its members from among the elite of the medical profession – from the Royal Colleges and the BMA. While noting general agreement over certain fundamental issues, they distinguished different possible lines of development largely in terms of methods of financing care and paying doctors. At one extreme they noted plans such as those of the BMA which simply advocated the extension of existing health services. At the other extreme were proposals to establish a full-time salaried medical service – such as those advanced by the SMA. Their own proposals can be located between these two extremes – the majority of the Commission's committees were opposed to the idea of a full-time salaried service and were of the opinion that team work, co-ordination, easier opportunities for post-graduate study, pension schemes and freedom from financial worry could be achieved without a wholly salaried service. Among the objections to such plans which they noted, without actually endorsing, were:

that the 'cold hand' of bureaucratic control, with the doctor acting under the orders of superior officers whether medical or lay, would be inimical to the wise and humane administration of a personal health service. The free-lance doctor turned civil servant . . . would suffer a diminution of his sense of personal responsibility for his patient and he would lose the spur to improved professional work and research. A profession of routine 'safe men' would be to the detriment of the country's health and medicine might cease to attract the proportion of first-class men it has attracted hitherto.[50]

What the Commission proposed was a range of three possible contractual arrangements for hospital doctors which included full-time salaried service with no private practice, full-time salaried employment with the right to undertake a limited amount of private practice within the hospital, and part-time salaried service with the freedom to engage in private practice both inside and outside the hospital. It made no proposals to merge the voluntary and public hospital systems, but did recommend that public grants be made to voluntary hospitals in order to enable them to offer the same salary scales as hospitals in the public system. They recognised that 'It is undesirable that in a unified scheme the important differences that prevail today between voluntary and council hospitals should persist',[51] but unification did not imply a complete merging of the hospital systems. They envisaged that the bulk of the population would finance their hospital care through regionally organised contributory schemes and for those whose incomes placed them above the limits of these schemes, they recommended provident insurance schemes.

National Health Insurance coverage was to be extended to the dependents of insured workers and it was proposed that benefits should include consultant, specialist and laboratory services. Regional health authorities, serving population units of at least 500,000 were to be introduced and these would establish health centres which would help to counteract the isolation of general practitioners. Apart from their income from a limited amount of private practice, GPs would be paid through the National Health Insurance scheme. In addition to a basic salary, the Commission proposed that they should receive extra payments on the basis of special qualifications and length of service, a capitation fee for the number of patients on their list, and fees for extraordinary services not covered by National Health Insurance. For those GPs who would be paid through public funds, the sales of practices was to be discontinued — an inducement to working in the public sphere.

Hardly a radical document, the Commission's report did, nevertheless, envisage a considerable extension of the state's function in providing health care for a majority of the population and did accept that a large proportion of the profession would receive the bulk of their remuneration from salaried service. But it could not accept the loss of rights to private practice, the incorporation of voluntary hospitals into the public system and the financing of hospital care through National Health Insurance or some other public scheme. It may have been clinging to symbols of freedom and it was, no doubt, unwilling to relinquish the most remunerative form of practice. Writing of the BMA's initial opposition to universal coverage, Forsyth comments that 'A cynic would interpret this as meaning that the BMA wanted to insure doctors against the patient's inability to pay rather than insure patients against the high cost of medical services'.[52] Such a cynical response to the proposals of the Medical Planning Commission might also be appropriate. But whether or not the proposals thus served the interests of the profession, they did involve a considerable expansion of state medical services.

Eckstein sees the report of the Commission as marking the height — short lived, yet intense — of reformist zeal in the profession.[53] Certainly, after 1942, the official position of the profession changed, but if for the moment, instead of looking forwards, we look back to 1920, we see that the proposals of the Commission bore marked similarities to those of the Consultative Council on Medical and Allied Services. The Council, appointed in 1919 by Addison, the first Minister of Health, also drew its membership from the elite of the profession. Yet despite such composition, the resulting Dawson Report has been seen by many as a visionary document — as 'one of the founding documents of the National Health Service', 'a guiding star', 'an immensely influential document' containing 'radical reforms'.[54] The terms of reference of the Council were to 'consider and make recommendations as to the scheme or schemes requisite for the systematised provision of such forms of medical and allied services as should in the opinion of the Council be available for the inhabitants of a given area'.[55] But despite the positive reception accorded to its report by the BMA and the press, the government took no action and the Council ceased to meet on a formal basis.

The report envisaged national health services 'available for all classes of the community' which emphasised both preventive and curative care. Apart from individual or some form of group practice, it proposed the introduction of Primary Health Centres from which domiciliary services would be provided by general practitioners and nurses and in which patients could receive short term institutional care. The staff of the centre would be complemented by visiting consultants and specialists. Diagnostic facilities for midwifery would be provided and community services such as prenatal care and examinations and treatment of school children would be located at the centre. These centres were to be supported by Secondary Health Centres which would serve a largely consultative function. Staffed mainly by consultants and specialists, they would take difficult cases and cases needing specialised treatment or equipment which had been referred by the Primary Health Centres. Ideally, they would be linked to teaching hospitals with medical schools. As far as the hospital system was concerned, rather than recommending a merging of voluntary and public hospitals, the Council advocated grants in aid for work done by the voluntary hospitals.

The Council was divided on the issue of how services were to be financed. Some members favoured the provision of services which were free at the time of use, with revenues presumably coming from taxation or insurance payments, but the majority felt that 'this course would impose a heavy burden on public funds'. They were of the opinion that whereas preventive services should be publicly financed because 'their relation to the individual is less obvious and personal', curative care is a 'direct personal concern' and should be paid for at least in part by the patient. They saw such costs as being met by 'some method of insurance', but it is not clear whether they meant National Health Insurance or insurance similar to that provided by contributory schemes and friendly societies. So while they did consider an expansion of state medical services, the range of public provisions which they envisaged, is not altogether clear. Similarly, the Council's position on the payment of doctors is vague. It opposed the idea of a full-time salaried service on the grounds that this would tend 'to discourage initiative, to diminish the sense of responsibility, and to encourage mediocrity',[56] but it did not elaborate on possible forms of part-time salaried service or other methods of payment.

Generally the report has been seen as forward looking and it contained many proposals in common with those in more radical plans for change. Indeed, many areas of agreement can be identified in the various proposals which were issued from the twenties to the early forties. What was debated was the extent of future state involvement in the health sector — whether or not there would be universal provision of public care; whether the profession would be employed in the public service on a full or part-time basis; what form their payments would assume, and whether a single public hospital system would be formed. Among the more radical conceptions of the future were the proposals of the Labour Party's Advisory Committee on Public Health, the SMA, Medical Planning Research and the 'Special Commissioner' appointed by *Lancet*.

Radical Proposals

The 1919 memorandum of the Advisory Committee on Public Health called for the reorganisation of the 'whole mechanism of medical care' rather than piecemeal change, though it did see the actual process of change as being gradual. It proposed a universal, comprehensive state medical service organised around health centres. Because of the problems the voluntary hospitals were facing, because 'a dual hospital system is bound to create difficulties and cause waste and over-lapping', and since 'medical aid and hospital accommodation should be the right of every citizen, and no one should be asked to accept them as charity',[57] it advocated the merging of the voluntary and public hospital systems. All doctors would be employed on a full-time salaried basis. It justified the universal and comprehensive nature of a state medical service on the basis that health is a national concern and the nation should collectively seek to preserve it. Any service catering to the poor alone, it argued, would inevitably be as inefficient and un-popular as Poor Law services had been. It pointed out that the rising costs of care were beyond the means of the majority of people — 'Many a patient has lost his life through trying to save a doctor's bill'[58] — and that as the service presently operated, middle class patients were excluded from institutional treatment.

The policy statement issued by the SMA in 1933 also proposed a universal comprehensive health service organised around health centres.[59] The services would be locally administered but nationally organised under the Ministry of Health and they would be available at no cost to all patients. Doctors were to be employed on a full-time salaried basis. A 'complete and co-ordinated hospital system' was seen to be a necessary element in the ideal medical service, yet the plans did not include a proposal to incorporate the voluntary hospitals into the public sector — the strongest recommendation was that no more volun-tary hospitals be founded unless the Ministry of Health considered them to be essential. However, the proposals did recommend the removal of all charges for care in public hospitals, with the anticipated consequence that:

the present financial difficulties of the voluntary hospitals will be increased. Those who are responsible for their management and have the good of the community at heart will see the need for a unified hospital system, and will desire increasing co-operation with the Municipal Hospitals and will be willing, it is hoped, to permit the local Public Health Committee to take over the management of their hospitals, so that they may be administered as part of the Municipal system.[60]

Somewhat more cautious proposals were advanced by the 'Special Commissioner' (Dr Stephen Taylor) appointed by *Lancet*.[61] In his plans for the reform of the hospital system, Taylor did not foresee the creation of a universal, comprehensive, national health service, free at the time of use for all patients. What he advocated was the extension of National Health Insurance to the dependents of workers (in order to reduce demands on outpatient departments) and that patients should either contribute according to their means to the costs of their hospital care or else be covered by some form of compulsory graded hospital insurance. Recognising that 'the great middle and upper-middle classes ask for and have a right to receive specialist and hospital treatment within their means',[62] he suggested that there might be private consulting clinics attached to the main outpatient centres, while the very rich 'who demand medical treatment at exorbitant prices' could still be served by private consultants and private nursing homes.[63] But he did propose the formation of a statutory National Hospital Corporation which would take over all hospitals and be responsible for the national co-ordination of a regionally organised hospital system. He also envisaged that the majority of the medical staff would be employed on a whole-time salaried basis.

The last of the series of reports issued within the profession was the Interim General Report of Medical Planning Research — a group which had been formed to give young doctors a stronger voice in the debates over the reorganisation of the health services.[64] Its report, published in *Lancet*, addressed broad social issues which it saw as appropriate for the post-war period — population policy, the productive capacity of the country, the problem of poverty etc. — and in so doing it advocated a comprehensive social security scheme, government intervention in the industrial structure 'for a planned economy', and, to cope with urban development problems, the transfer of all land and buildings 'into the ownership or at least full control of the state'. As far as the health care system was concerned, it envisaged a comprehensive and universal social security scheme to which all would contribute, though people earning over £500 per annum would have the chance to opt out of one-eighth of their contributions and forego any medical benefits. Under the scheme, pensions, unemployment benefits, family allowances, burial allowances, maternity and sickness benefits and all necessary forms of health care would be provided. Payments into the scheme would be graded in relation to income and wage earners would pay no more than 8 to 10 per cent of their income. It also recommended that people be given the opportunity to pay higher contributions and in return receive extra privacy in hospital treatment and exemptions from clinical demonstrations. With an even higher contribution, people would be entitled to increased benefits and pensions.

It advocated the establishment of health centres and the unification of the hospital system, with voluntary hospitals being incorporated into the public system. Medical staff were to be salaried and in addition to their basic salary general practitioners would receive capitation fees and fees for special services. It was proposed that the central authority for this unified health service should be a corporate body rather than a Department of State. A National Health Corporation — similar in status to the BBC — was favoured because it was less likely to be bureaucratic and hierarchical (thus lacking the rigidity and strictures on professional freedoms which these characteristics might imply), more likely to be free from political pressures and able to engage in longer term planning than any health service organised directly under a Ministry of Health.

These reports which I have labelled as 'radical' are not so labelled simply because they favour state intervention in the health sector, for each of the major reports issued during the inter-war years proposed an extension of the state's function in financing and organising health services. They are distinctive insofar as they favour a universal and comprehensive national health service, the establishment of which would involve the merging of voluntary and public hospitals into a single public system, and the employment of the medical profession on a full-time salaried basis. But these more radical proposals for reform were not voices 'crying in the wilderness' for change — they bore many similarities with more cautious proposals and it is important to recognise that a considerable portion of the profession, including its leaders, favoured an extensive public medical care service which was at least partially salaried.

Yet this apparent consensus in published documents does not mean that the profession as a whole was relatively complacent about the course of change and that it accepted, with few reservations, an extension of state functions. Indeed, the correspondence pages of *Lancet* and the *British Medical Journal* belie any such conclusions. Despite official pronouncements, some doctors were fearful of the effects of an increase in the state's responsibility in providing health care.

Responses to the Proposals

The responses to just a few of the reports help to convey the thoughts and feelings of individual physicians. In letters commenting on the plan advanced by the 'Special Commissioner' appointed by *Lancet*, many correspondents voiced a considerable amount of support for the details and principles of the proposals, but others referred to it as a 'horrific nightmare', 'totalitarian' in conception and placing upon the hospitals 'the fetters of large scale organisation'.[65] One correspondent asked: 'Is this what the war is for? I thought it was to fight against methods of this sort'; others thought that 'competition and individual initiative are destroyed' and that 'liberty of action is restricted'. But many of the letters congratulated *Lancet* on the 'excellent plan' and considered it to be 'admirable' and a 'realistic report' of the situation and future of British hospitals, which 'deserves the thanks of the whole profession'. One correspondent wrote:

> I can only congratulate you and your special commissioner on the courage you have shown in storming the citadel. I have waited for the howls of wrath and indignation from the old gentlemen and from all the vested interests, and have been surprised at the ineffective bleat of protest from those who feel themselves so much assailed . . . one finds mainly criticism of such detail as to whether half-time service is better than whole-time for consultants, with vague generalisations about inheritance of freedom and traditions of service mixed with disgruntlement arising from the EMS.[66]

Letters responding to the ideas of the Medical Planning Commission also indicate a range of views within the profession.[67] Some argued that the 'freedom of the doctor and patient would disappear', that such proposals would 'deprive the medical profession of its traditional professional freedom', and that 'Collective medicine may suit some countries but it is unsuitable for this England of ours'. But many others were supportive or even critical of the report in that it did not go far enough. One correspondent, arguing that more attention be devoted to preventive medicine, education and the improvement of working and housing conditions, thought that the medical profession had failed to give an intelligent lead to the public and urged 'This is our moment; let us have vision beyond tomorrow and build worthily for the future',[68] Another, claiming that the Commissioners had failed to address the problem of underdoctored areas, commented that the report 'seems to have been written by gentlemen wearing professional blinkers which have entirely shut out the public interest and forced them to concentrate on their own.[69]

In the negative responses to the various reports, we see some evidence for traditional images of conflict between the profession and the state — of the threat which state intervention is seen to present to professional freedoms (and freedom *per se* for some correspondents). But these were not the most common sentiments and most physicians appear to have recognised a need for change and for the state's assumption of responsibility in organising and financing a unified national health service. By 1942, the majority of the profession was urging change:

> The whole profession seemed to be in a reformist heat. It is said that late that year it was impossible to stage a debate on the desirability of a comprehensive State Medical service in one of the London teaching hospitals because no one could be found to oppose such a service.[70]

Yet as we have seen, this concern with comprehensive reform was by no means a recent one — as it was in the union movement — similar issues had been debated, though with less fervour and urgency perhaps, since the 1920s. No doubt Somerville Hastings of the SMA had echoed the sentiments of many when he argued that he saw two courses as being open to the profession:

> it could wait and do nothing, and then the politicians would suddenly wake up and would inflict some incomplete and undigested scheme like the panel or something worse; or it could see what was coming and try to mould public opinion, so that when the change did come a service would be formed which would be advantageous both to the science of medicine and to the public generally.[71]

Quite obviously, the profession pursued the latter option, but in so doing, did not fight against state intervention.

The most immediate question which springs from these observations is that of why the profession was amenable to further state intervention in the health sector. For this does not coincide with our usual images of the profession's attitude towards socialised medicine. Then also, given such attitudes, why was it that the profession appears to have completely reversed its position by opposing the government's proposals for a national health service?

State Medical Services and Professional Interests

Many discussions of the medical profession see it as a conservative force which reluctantly accepts change and vehemently opposes proposals to introduce any form of socialised medicine. This perceived opposition is seen to be founded in the profession's desire to preserve autonomy and a belief that state intervention in the health sector will erode professional freedoms by intruding in the doctor-patient relationship, increasing the level of consumer control and bureaucratising the social context of medicine. Both patients and physicians are seen to suffer from the mediocrity of practice which flows from such controls. While such opposition may be common, it obviously does not characterise the stance of the profession in Britain during the twenties, thirties and early forties. How can we explain the pressures for change and the promotion of more extensive state medical services?

Given that physicians' experience of the health services was broader and richer in nature than those who had only selective contact with them as patients, and that this experience heightened their awareness of problems, it is hardly surprising that they were in the forefront of pressures for reform. The services provided far from ideal conditions in which to practice and it was in the interests of the profession to seek to correct those problems which directly affected them — inadequate and out-dated facilities; financial restrictions; the increasing difficulty of private patients in meeting medical bills; the inadequacies of contract practice; demarcation disputes between general practitioners, consultants and hospitals; the high capital outlay necessary to set up practice and other similar problems. With its knowledge and interest in improving conditions of work, it should be no surprise that the profession was creating an awareness of a need for change and advancing proposals for reform. But whether we adopt an image of the profession as altruistic and service oriented or as self-serving, it is unusual that the proposals for change should involve a significant extension of state medical services, for the profession is typically seen to reject this on the basis of the negative consequences for *both* patient and physician.

One important feature of medical services in pre-war Britain which helps to explain the response of the profession is the fact that no strong private interests had developed in the health sector. Private insurance schemes were generally small and locally organised and in no position to act as powerful pressure groups on either the profession or the state. Neither were they in a position to assume any responsibility for the co-ordination and financing of health services on a national basis. This absence of strong private interests helps to explain the fact that the profession advocated a publicly planned national health service: no other options existed. As Abel-Smith comments:

> the prepayment agencies in Britain were unbusinesslike, ineffectively co-ordinated and run by persons without power or influence. They were swept into the background without antagonising any important section of opinion. If the large profit-making insurance interests had ever entered the hospital field, the replacement of 'voluntary' prepayment with a scheme based on taxation and compulsory 'contributions' would have been less easily accomplished. [72]

The only legitimate institutional framework within which planning could occur was that of the state, and precedents for such had already been established. More importantly, these incursions of the state into the health sector had not threatened the interests of physicians. National Health Insurance had served the material interests of the profession and a national health service promised to further improve the financial situation of physicians. Contract practice and the outpatient departments of voluntary hospitals had been exerting a depressing effect on the income of general practitioners, especially those practicing in working class areas. National Health Insurance had partly resolved this problem, but, as Forsyth points out, 'even in the late 1930s many GPs still earned relatively low incomes: of those between 40 and 49 years of age almost two thirds earned less than £1,300 per annum and nearly one quarter earned less than £700'. [73] Johnson suggests that 'practitioners less favoured by the fee system will be likely to form a pressure group within the occupation seeking some modification of the producer-consumer relationship'. [74] The National Health Insurance scheme had proved to be a financially acceptable modification, one which the profession was ready to extend. Moreover, state medical services which employed physicians on a partly salaried basis promised to shield them against unpaid medical bills while preserving their rights to treat wealthier patients on a private basis; the fact that it was quite common for doctors to employ debt collectors, suggests that such a 'shield' would be welcome. [75] Specialists stood to gain much from a part-time salaried service; the early years of financial sacrifice would disappear, some uniformity of payment would be introduced, their earnings would be independent of GP referrals, and they could afford to delegate less interesting and less specialised work to juniors.[76]

Quite apart from the financial benefits which accrued to the profession, it seems to have experienced few burdensome restrictions of its autonomy. At least, this is what we might infer from the willingness of the BMA in 1917 to suggest the inclusion of dependents in the National Health Insurance scheme. Certainly, employment in public medical services seemed preferable to other forms of contract practice. Apart from the financial benefits which had accrued to the profession, state intervention in the health sector had posed minimal threats to the autonomy which the profession enjoyed in the practice of medicine. Referring to the National Health Insurance scheme, the Medical Planning Commission noted that: 'Its medical service contains features which have proved to be essentially sound such as free choice of doctor, the minimum of interference by the state, and the central negotiation of terms and conditions of service'.[77]

To argue that the extension of state medical services was perceived as no real threat to professional autonomy (and thus accepted) is to leave open the issue of whose interests were being served in the formulation of plans for a national health service. To what extent can the profession's proposals for reform be interpreted as an instance of its service orientation or of its self-serving nature? Insofar as autonomy is necessary in order for physicians to provide patients with the best available medical care, then obviously the interests of patients will be met by the preservation of this autonomy. Yet insofar as this autonomy is guarded in order to preserve the power and prestige of the profession, it is self-serving. If we accept the profession's models of illness and appropriate health care, then there is no necessary conflict here — no sense in which patient and professional interests are fundamentally opposed. But if, on the other hand, we recognise the social and political nature of such medical models, then an objective conflict of interests has to be admitted, and, the desire of the profession to retain the degree of autonomy it enjoyed, must be seen as serving professional interests and not those of patients.

In recent years several writers have questioned the efficacy of medicine, drawn attention to the political basis of the profession's 'medical model' and argued that this serves the interests of the profession by providing the bases on which it claims power and autonomy.[78] Others have also emphasised the manner in which professional definitions of sickness and health serve the process of capital accumulation.[79] Not surprisingly, the proposals for reform which the profession advanced, raised no such issues. Minimal emphasis was placed upon the social bases of illness and while there were brief references to the importance of preventive medicine, these seldom showed any appreciation of the links between the level and nature of illness and the social organisation of British society. Though sometimes fearful of the bureaucratic and hierarchical organisation which might stem from state intervention, the profession's desire to further rationalise the organisation of health services implied greater bureaucratisation and a clarification of professional hierarchies. There was little discussion of different modes of allocation of professional responsibilities and of extending greater responsibility to para-professionals. Similarly, there was no debate over the efficacy of medicine and the desirability of technological developments in the health sector. While it may be totally unrealistic to expect the profession to have been grappling with such issues, it is important to recognise that such issues *are* open to debate and that professional definitions of illness and appropriate care are not wholly founded on scientific expertise, but are social creations. The power and autonomy of the profession is founded in such definitions and the scientific rationale which is claimed for them. But they serve patients' interests only as these are defined by the profession. Insofar as proposals for change remained within the bounds of these definitions then they served the interests of physicians and presented health as an issue of access to professional care.

My emphasis thus far has been on the way in which socialised medicine appeared to serve the interests of the medical profession. However, the opposition of the profession to government plans for the NHS appears to deny the validity of this argument. This opposition started in 1943 when the plans of Ernest Brown, the Minister of Health, became known, and it continued even beyond the passage of the National Health Service Act in 1946.[80] As Eckstein notes, 'As soon as the Government became serious about reforming the medical system, a sort of nameless fear of what might ensue gripped the profession's representatives'.[81] Yet this opposition need not necessarily be interpreted as a rejection of socialised medicine *per se*. As we have already seen, opinions varied within the profession concerning such issues as salaried service, universal coverage and the merging of voluntary and public hospital systems. Responses to the government plans also varied; among the more receptive were younger physicians, those already employed in public medical services, doctors with experience in the armed forces, and specialists. In other words, physicians who had some familiarity with the impact of non-medical organisation on medical practice and those who were in less financially lucrative situations were more likely to approve the government plans. We cannot speak of the response of the profession as a whole, for opinions differed. Yet the opinons which were voiced most loudly, and which seemed to represent the profession, were those of the leaders of the BMA[82] — older men, with experience largely in general practice; men who had lived through and probably forgotten the years of financial sacrifices and insecurity which young GPs and specialists experienced in establishing a practice and a reputation. So while there was quite widespread opposition to the government's proposals, this often focused on specific details and was certainly not as strong as the leaders of the BMA had hoped and insufficient for them to organise a boycott of the NHS.

We can further understand the opposition of the profession as a response to the fact that once the government took the initiative in re-organising the health services, the profession's sense of control over the process of change was lost. Here again, I would argue that the profession was not rejecting the concept of socialised medicine *per se*, but rather that it was opposing the manner in which the plans for the service were being formulated. It is reasonable to assume that the profession expected to play a part in designing a national health service. Physicians' involvement in drawing up earlier proposals for change and their representation on government bodies concerned with the reorganisation of the health services — appointments to the Consultative Council on Medical and Allied Services, the opportunity to make representations to the Royal Commission on National Health Insurance and the participation of physicians in the establishment of the Emergency Medical Service, for example — would undoubtedly lead to the expectation of some involvement in the planning of a new service. The initial opposition to National Health Insurance, which had largely resulted from the lack of consultation with the profession, would lead physicians to suppose that the government would proceed more carefully this time round and more fully involve them in the process of planning. Yet no such expectations were met. The BMA proposed that the issue should be the subject of a Royal Commission — in which its views would no doubt be represented — but this idea was never taken up. Though Willink, as Minister of Health, consulted with the profession, after the Labour victory in the 1945 General Election and the appointment of Aneurin Bevan as Minister of Health, all forms of negotiation ceased and the National Health Service Act was passed without significant input from the profession. Insofar as the profession was excluded from the process of planning, opposition became important as part of a bargaining strategy, as a means of gaining concessions from the state.

The opposition which did exist can also be viewed as something more than a bargaining strategy. The exclusion of the profession from the formulation of plans highlights the fact that it is not ultimately autonomous. Professional autonomy is not absolute but is granted by the state.[83] But the nature of this relationship between state and profession is seldom revealed; only in the process of the state changing the social organisation of medical practice is the objective character of this relationship apparent. It is in the light of the essential conflict arising from the subordination of the profession that we may understand the opposition of the profession. Though this was directed at the content of state proposals, it may in part be seen as a means of challenging the form of the relationship between state and profession. It was not so much an opposition to incursions on professional autonomy as opposition to the fact that the profession is not ultimately autonomous.

Conclusion

It appears to be overly simplistic to assume that socialised medicine is necessarily a threat to professional autonomy and thus inimical to the interests of the profession. At least in this historical setting, there is evidence to suggest that the bulk of the medical profession favoured some extension of state medical services and played an important part in shaping the debate over reform. In the various proposals issued by different branches of the profession, the main concern was with rationalising the organisation and funding of health care. There is little evidence that the profession was largely concerned with improving the access to care of working class patients, for many other problems also occupied its attention and comprehensive reform was seen as being necessary in order to achieve a more rationally ordered and efficient health care system.

The extension of state medical services promised to serve the interests of the profession by rationalising the health care system, improving facilities, increasing levels of remuneration, reducing the insecurity and financial burdens of the early years of practice and allowing consultants to more narrowly specialise in their areas of interest. Insofar as there was opposition to the government proposals for the NHS, this was strongest within the leadership of the profession, and, apart from being a convenient bargaining strategy, this opposition may be viewed as a response to the exclusion of physicians from the planning of the new service. While the profession may have played a large part in shaping the debate over reform, and though socialised medicine may be seen as serving the profession's interests, the state's assumption of responsibility for the creation of the NHS, highlighted the dependency of the profession on the state for the degree of autonomy which it enjoyed.

Notes

1. Rodney M. Coe, *Sociology of Medicine* (McGraw-Hill, London, 1970), pp. 331-2; Elliott A. Krause, *Power and Illness: The Political Sociology of Health and Medical Care* (Elsevier, New York, 1977), pp. 26-30; M.W. Susser and W. Watson, *Sociology in Medicine*, 2nd edn (Oxford University Press, London, 1971), pp. 237-275.

2. Vicente Navarro, 'The Industrialization of Fetishism or the Fetishism of Industrialization: A Critique of Ivan Illich', *Social Science and Medicine*, vol. 9 (1975), p. 358.

3. For example, the threatened boycotts in Britain in 1911 and 1948 and the strikes in Saskatchewan and Quebec in 1962 and 1970.

4. For an example of the way in which state intervention is seen to threaten professional autonomy see Friedson's discussion of medicine in the USA, Eliot Friedson, *Profession of Medicine: A Study of the Sociology of Applied Knowledge* (Harper and Row, New York, 1970), pp. 25-33. A discussion of the conflicts between professional and bureaucratic authority can be found in Susser and Watson, *Sociology in Medicine*, pp. 237-75.

5. Eliot Friedson, *Profession of Medicine: A Study of the Sociology of Applied Knowledge* (Harper and Row, New York, 1970).

6. Ibid., p. 25.

7. Jeanne L. Brand, *Doctors and the State: The British Medical Profession and Government Action in Public Health, 1870-1912* (The Johns Hopkins Press, Baltimore, 1965), pp. 230, 236; Gordon Forsyth, *Doctors and State Medicine: A Study of the British Health Service* (Pitman Medical Publishing Company Ltd, London, 1966), p. 6.

8. Richard M. Titmuss, 'Health' in Morris Ginsberg (ed.), *Law and Opinion in England in the 20th Century* (University of California Press, Berkeley, 1959), p. 312.

9. Ruth G. Hodgkinson, *The Origins of the National Health Service* (The Wellcome Historical Medical Library, London, 1967), p. 683.

10. Ibid.

11. Ibid., p. 450.

12. Brand, *Doctors and the State*, p. 229.

13. The Labour Party, Memoranda Prepared by the Advisory Committee on Public Health, I, *The Organisation of the Preventative and Curative Medical Services and Hospital and Laboratory Systems Under a Ministry of Health* (The Labour Party, London, 1919).

14. Ministry of Health, Consultative Council on Medical and Allied Services, *Interim Report on the Future Provision of Medical and Allied Services* (HMSO,

London, 1920).

15. British Medical Association, *Proposals for a General Medical Service for the Nation* (British Medical Association, London, 1929); ibid., *A General Medical Service for the Nation* (British Medical Association, London, 1938).

16. Socialist Medical Association, *A Socialised Medical Service* (Socialist Medical Association, London, 1933).

17. 'A Plan for British Hospitals', *Lancet*, ii (1939), pp. 945-51.

18. Medical Planning Commission, 'Draft Interim Report, *British Medical Journal*, vol. 1 (1942), pp. 743-53.

19. Medical Planning Research, 'Interim General Report', *Lancet* , ii (1942), pp. 599-622.

20. *British Medical Journal*, Supplement, i (1942), pp. 1-98.

21. The Labour Party, *Organisation of Preventative and Curative Medical Services*, p. 1.

22. Ibid., p. 2.

23. Ibid.

24. Ibid., p. 6.

25. *British Medical Journal*, Supplement, i (1942), p. 1.

26. Medical Planning Research, 'Interim General Report', p. 618.

27. Ibid.

28. *Lancet*, i (1934), p. 792.

29. Ministry of Health,Consultative Council on Medical and Allied Services, *Interim Report*, pp. 15-16.

30. The Labour Party, *Organisation of Preventative and Curative Medical Services*, p. 5.

31. 'A Plan for British Hospitals', p. 946.

32. British Medical Association, *General Medical Service*, p. 6.

33. Ibid., p. 3.

34. Ibid., p. 7.

35. Medical Planning Commission, 'Draft Interim Report', p. 743.

36. 'A Plan for British Hospitals', p. 947.

37. Medical Planning Research, 'Interim General Report', p. 618.

38. Socialist Medical Association, *The Socialist Programme for Health* (Socialist Medical Association, London, 1943), p. 7.

39. Medical Planning.Commission, 'Draft Interim Report', p. 744.

40. *British Medical Journal*, Supplement, i (1942), p. 1.

41. *Lancet*, ii (1939), p. 315.

42. Ibid., p. 331.

43. 'A Plan for British Hospitals', p. 945.

44. Michael Foote, *Aneurin Bevan: Volume Two, 1945-1960* (Davis-Poynter, London, 1973), p. 103.

45. Ibid.

46. British Medical Association, *General Medical Service*, p. 3.

47. *Lancet*, ii (1942), p. 345.

48. Ibid.

49. Medical Planning Commission, 'Draft Interim Report'.

50. Ministry of Health, Consultative Council on Medical and Allied Services, *Interim Report*, p. 746.

51. Ibid., p. 750.

52. Forsyth, *Doctors and State Medicine*, p. 15.

53. Harry Eckstein, *The English Health Service: Its Origins, Structure and Achievements* (Harvard University Press, Cambridge, Mass., 1958), p. 118.

54. Brian Watkins, *Documents on Health and Social Services: 1834 to the Present Day* (Methuen, London, 1975), pp. 111-12.

55. Ministry of Health, Consultative Council on Medical and Allied Services, *Interim Report*, p. 5.

56. Ibid., p. 11.

57. The Labour Party, *Organisation of Preventative and Curative Medical Services*, p. 5.

58. Ibid., p. 6.

59. Socialist Medical Association, *A Socialised Medical Service*.

60. Ibid., p. 19.

61. 'A Plan for British Hospitals'.

62. Ibid., p. 949.

63. Ibid.

64. Medical Planning Research, 'Interim General Report'.

65. For letters in response to the plans of the 'Special Commissioner', see *Lancet*, ii (1939), pp. 1002-3, 1043-6, 1093-7, 1141-4, 1193-5, 1239-41, 1285-7, 1292. Lord Horder summarised the debate in ibid., pp. 1342-3.

66. Ibid., p . 1141.

67. For comments on the proposals of the Medical Planning Commission see *Lancet*, ii (1942), pp. 23-4, 53, 84, 112, 294.

68. Ibid., p. 23.

69. Ibid., p. 112.

70. Eckstein, *The English Health Service*, p. 122.

71. *Lancet*, i (1932), p. 839.

72. Brian Abel-Smith, *The Hospitals 1800-1948* (Heinemann, London, 1964), p. 499.

73. Forsyth, *Doctors and State Medicine*, p. 26.

74. Terence J. Johnson, *Professions and Power* (Macmillan, London, 1972), p. 59.

75. Forsyth, *Doctors and State Medicine*, p. 26.

76. Ibid., p. 23.

77. Medical Planning Commission, 'Draft Interim Report', p. 747.

78. Hans Peter Dreitzel, *The Social Organization of Health* (Macmillan, New York, 1971); Friedson, *Profession of Medicine*; Ivan Illich, *Limits to Medicine* (McClelland and Stewart, Toronto, 1976); Martin Rossdale, 'Health in a Sick Society', *New Left Review*, no. 34 (1965), pp. 82-91.

79. Marc Renaud, 'On the Structural Constraints to State Intervention in Health', *International Journal of Health Services*, vol. 5, no. 4 (1975), pp. 559-71; Terence Johnson, 'Professions, Class and the State', Paper presented at the Annual Meetings of the Canadian Sociology and Anthropology Association, Quebec City, 1976.

80. For a fuller discussion of the profession's response see Eckstein, *The English Health Service*; Forsyth, *Doctors and State Medicine*; Arthur J. Willcocks, *The Creation of the National Health Service* (Routledge and Kegan Paul, London, 1967).

81. Eckstein, *The English Health Service*, p. 143.

82. Ibid., p. 151.

83. Friedson, *Profession of Medicine*; Navarro, 'The Industrialization of Fetishism'.

6 THE INTRODUCTION OF THE NHS

We have already seen that there is little evidence to suggest that the NHS was a response to class conflict. Working class patients were not singularly disadvantaged in their access to care and representatives of the organised working class were not pressing for comprehensive reform of the health services until a relatively late stage in the debate over reorganisation. Rather, I have argued that the NHS was an effort to rationalise the organisation and financing of medical services. This argument is lent support by several observations. Apart from the problems which working class and middle class patients faced in obtaining adequate care, there were many other deficiencies in the organisation and funding of health services and these became increasingly severe during the twenties and thirties. Though the Trades Union Congress and the Labour Party played a part in drawing attention to these problems, it was groups representing different branches of the medical profession which recognised the fullest range of problems and were most involved in defining a need for comprehensive reform. They played an important role in shaping the debate over reform and saw some extension of state medical services as being the means whereby a rational, efficient and financially viable health service might be created.[1]

This theme of rationalisation is also evident in statements made on behalf of both the Conservative and Labour parties during the period when plans for a national health service were being formulated. The Beveridge Report of 1942 received a warm reception from both parties and from the public.[2] Debates in the House of Commons indicate that the principles underlying Beveridge's recommendations were generally welcomed and of those members of the public surveyed by the British Institute of Public Opinion, 88 per cent favoured the idea of a comprehensive medical service — it was one of the most popular recommendations.[3] In the House of Commons, the social insurance proposals were understood, at least implicitly, in class terms; their importance in guaranteeing a minimum standard of living, providing a measure of security and contributing to post-war reconstruction were acknowledged. But the proposals for a public medical service were presented somewhat differently and were viewed in the context of the Government's ongoing concern with reform of the health care system. Sir John Anderson, Lord

President of the Council, speaking to the Beveridge Report on behalf of the Government, said that

> The Government welcome this conception of a reorganised and comprehensive health service. The conception does not necessarily spring from the particular social security structure with which the Report is concerned. It is, in fact, the consummation of a general process which has been going on steadily, if piecemeal, under successive Governments for a great many years, a constant movement to improve and make more comprehensive the personal health services.[4]

He recognised the importance of providing ready access to different types of medical care, of making the fullest use of existing resources, securing co-operation between the various units providing care and establishing responsibility for a 'full and efficient' service. Class inequalities in health and access to care were not emphasised. The major focus was on rationalisation:

> with the war and the chances of post-war reconstruction there is an opportunity to pull together many of the loose strands of the last 20 or 30 years, and build up the whole service on rational lines until it justifies in every sense the word 'comprehensive'.[5]

This same theme can also be identified in the statement made to the House of Commons by Willink, the Conservative Minister of Health, at the time his White Paper was issued. He argued that the plans laid out in the White Paper 'are those which the Government believe to be best calculated to achieve an efficient and comprehensive National Health Service'.[6] He added that

> This is no scheme for giving charity to individuals or State help to particular classes or groups. This scheme does not concern itself with poverty or wealth. It is a plan to raise national health to a higher plane and keep it there, and to use the nation's full resources to raise it even higher.[7]

Two years later, Aneurin Bevan, as Labour Minister of Health, moved the second reading of the National Health Service Bill. In his comments and in the ensuing debate, there was a more marked concern with the problems working class patients experienced in obtaining health care.[8] These problems were traced to the deficiencies of the National Health Insurance scheme, its limited coverage and the uneven distribution of facilities and manpower. Yet though this was a more dominant theme than in earlier years, it was but one of several concerns. The main goal was to build an efficient health service by co-ordinating the units providing care, reducing the isolation of doctors, improving the facilities in which they worked, redistributing services and replacing the many small hospitals throughout the country with larger, more efficient hospitals. Efficiency was emphasised above all else. Indeed, both parties placed considerable emphasis on the need to create a rational, efficient and nationally co-ordinated health service. There were differences between the parties, especially in the solutions they proposed to the problem of the voluntary hospitals, but there was an overwhelming consensus as to the need for an extensive state medical service.

There is therefore, much evidence to suggest that the NHS was directed at the rationalisation of the health services. It was assumed that the introduction of an efficient, nationally co-ordinated health service would improve the access to care of all classes. Moreover, it was argued that such improvements would 'raise national health to a higher plane'. In effect, health was seen to depend largely on patients' access to medical care. But what of the impact of the service? The common conceptions of the NHS portray it as a redistributive measure which gave working class patients easy access to medical care and which, for the first time, provided care on the basis of need rather than the ability to pay for treatment. How valid is such an assessment?

The Significance of the NHS for Working Class and Middle Class Patients

The changes which came with the introduction of the NHS had relatively little immediate impact on the actual delivery of medical care. It was some time before the redistribution of hospital and general practitioner services made itself felt and improvements in the quality of hospital and primary care were not always experienced immediately.[9] The majority of patients were likely to receive care from the same doctor and hospital, though they would have to consult their GP in order to be referred to a hospital. For the poor, used to consulting the outpatient department of a hospital for care, there was, therefore, a change in the pattern of obtaining care. For wealthier patients, used to paying for private care, there was the opportunity to receive treatment in former local authority and voluntary hospitals. But the major difference for most people was in the method of paying for treatment. Here, the financial benefits were certainly as significant for the middle class as for the working class patient, and these, together with the removal of the barrier to admission to the local authority and hospitals, convey the importance of the NHS for middle class families.

Just prior to the introduction of the NHS, many patients provided for their treatment through contributory or provident schemes. Working class patients belonged to contributory schemes which required only partial prepayment for care and which served those who were unable to pay the full costs of treatment. Families in the middle and upper classes who did not pay private fees whenever care was necessary, provided for their needs through provident insurance schemes which aimed to cover the full costs of care. The aged, unemployed and those who did not or could not make regular payments into such schemes had the right to free hospital treatment after a means test. Local authorities, through public assistance committees, made arrangements for the medical attention of the destitute. With the NHS, free care became a right of all citizens and so, inasmuch as there had been a stigma attached to receiving free care, this was removed. Even partial payments for treatment were a burden for many families close to destitution, and, therefore, the removal of the direct costs of treatment was welcomed by lower income families. But the benefits flowing from the NHS were not confined to working class families alone. We should consider for a moment the position of middle class families.

One neglected section of the population which was feeling the pinch of the increasing costs of care, was made up of families in middle income brackets. They were not eligible for charity care and the income limits operating in contributory schemes generally excluded them. They were private fee paying patients of general practitioners, and in the hospitals, they either paid the full cost of care whenever hospitalised or else guarded against such unanticipatable high bills by membership in a provident insurance scheme. They 'bore the brunt of neglect' in that they received no financial concessions in meeting their medical needs and, at the same time, indirectly subsidised the poor. The NHS brought them the first such concessions. The benefits which accrued to middle class families are illustrated by a business executive who recounts the freedom from worry over expenses of childbirth and any major illness in the family which came with the NHS,[10] and a middle class father of four children wrote, 'I can see that to middle class families, it is not just a benefit, but a necessity; the cost of living has risen so greatly since 1939 that private medical care would be another increasingly expensive burden.'[11] In introducing the NHS, the Minister of Health spoke of its special value to families in the middle and professional classes who had so often been 'hit cruelly hard by heavy surgical and medical fees which have a habit of coming at the wrong moment'.[12]

But the NHS did not only provide middle class patients with important financial benefits; it also secured their access to the mainstream of the hospital system. As we have already seen, prior to the introduction of the service, middle class families were generally unable to obtain care in the local authority and voluntary hospital systems. Instead, they were confined to smaller and less well equipped private hospitals and nursing homes. With the introduction of the new service, they were able to gain access to the often superior care available in the major hospitals.[13] At the same time, they secured the privilege of paying for private care in these hospitals, thus receiving benefits not available to NHS patients.[14] Those analyses which emphasise the benefits experienced by working class patients as a result of the introduction of the NHS fail to convey the importance of the service to middle class families. It was not a change which catered to the problems of the working class alone.

Access to Primary Care

Mechanic argues that 'the National Health Service demonstrates the possibility of providing a "reasonable" level of medical care . . . in terms of need rather than ability to pay'.[15] If, as he implies, the NHS was successful in improving the access to physician care of working class patients, we should be able to identify different rates of consultation by these patients before and after the introduction of the new service. Specifically, we would expect rates of consultation with physicians to be lowest among working class patients before 1948 and we would expect a rise in these rates after 1948 — a rise of such magnitude that working class patients started to make more frequent use of physician services than did middle class patients. Moreover, it is reasonable to expect this change in consultation rates to be most marked for working class women: while physician care was provided free for manual workers under National Health Insurance, their wives and children received charitable care or provided for their health needs through membership in schemes offered by friendly societies, doctors' clubs, etc. Thus the costs of obtaining care were somewhat higher for unemployed working class women and children than for working class men. This leads us to suppose that the removal of the direct costs of obtaining care which was effected by the NHS, would have a greater impact on the consultation rates of working class women than on those of their male counterparts. To what extent are these various expectations matched by data?

Unfortunately, there is little data on the use of physician services before 1948 and that which is available covers a period of relatively high employment — we know relatively little about patterns of consultation in periods of unemployment.[16] On the basis of the data which are available, it is not entirely clear that working class patients were disadvantaged in access to physician care prior to 1948. In one study of an industrial town, 93 per cent of the families indicated that they were getting adequate treatment before the introduction of the NHS[17] and *Survey of Sickness* data for January 1946 and for 1947 do not show consistently lower rates of consultation among working class patients.[18] Those for January 1946 do suggest that working class patients had less easy access to physicians than did middle class patients — while morbidity rates were lower than average for those in professional and managerial occupations, their rates of consultation with physicians were higher than average, and though morbidity rates were only slightly higher than average for clerical workers, their consultation rates were among the highest.[19] However, medical consultation rates for 1947, which are shown in Table 6.1, show a rough correspondence with morbidity rates and the apparent class bias indicated by the data for January 1946 is not evident. With the exception of agricultural workers, consultation rates tend to vary in the same manner as sickness, prevalence and incapacity rates.

Given such contradictory patterns, we can reach no firm conclusions about the access to care of patients of different social class — we just do not have sufficient data to indicate whether or not working class patients made less use of health services than their needs for care lead us to expect.[20]

Any assessment of the impact of the NHS is limited by the paucity of data on patterns of consultation before 1948. But, bearing in mind the limitations of such a comparison, if we compare data on rates of consultation with physicians for men and women in 1947, 1949 and 1951, we see only minor changes in patterns of use. Table 6.2 presents these data in relation to income. The rates for those in the lowest income category are higher than those for other income groups in each of the years. While there were no marked changes in morbidity rates (those for 1947 and 1951 are almost identical) the consultation rates for the two lowest income groups are higher in 1949 and 1951. For men in other income groups there are no marked differences in

Table 6.1: Mean Monthly Sickness, Prevalence and Incapacity Rates by Occupational Groups, Males, England and Wales, 1947

Occupational Group	Sickness Rate[a]	Prevalence Rate[b]	Incapacity Rate[c]	Medical Consultation Rate[d]
Professional and Managerial	58	101	56	29
Clerical	56	98	80	31
Operatives and other grades:				
Manufacturing	60	110	98	35
Transport and Public Service	57	98	98	37
Mining and Quarrying	69	133	182	51
Building and Roadmaking	56	96	81	27
Agriculture	53	91	80	23
Distributive	58	104	72	33
Other Industries	57	103	82	32
Total	61	114	106	39

Notes: a. The percentage of people reporting some illness or injury in a month.
 b. The number of illnesses or injuries in a month per 100 persons interviewed.
 c. The number of days off work or confined to the home in a month per 100 persons interviewed.
 d. The number of visits with a practitioner in a month per 100 persons interviewed.
Source: General Register Office, *The Survey of Sickness, 1943-52*, Studies in Medical and Population Subjects, no. 12 (HMSO, London, 1957), pp. 50-1.

consultation rates in 1947, but in 1949 and, more obviously in 1951, consultation rates decline as income increases. For women in these income categories there is a consistent increase in consultation rates with increasing income in 1947, no marked differences in 1949 and a steady decline in rates as income increases in 1951. These changing patterns of consultations may be a result of the increased availability of free care which achieved a closer correspondence between people's needs for care and their use of health services. But it is important to note that the increases are smaller for women than for men in the lowest income category. This is curious, seeing as it was working class women and not men, who had free general practitioner care extended to them in 1948. We might also note that while women experience somewhat higher morbidity than men, in the lower income groups their consultation rates are lower than those for men in each of the three years.[21]

When the consultations rates for males are analysed by occupation rather than income, there is no evidence of a consistently greater increase in rates for manual workers than for those men in professional,

Table 6.2: Mean Monthly Medical Consultation Rates by Sex and Income Group of Chief Wage Earner, 1947 and 1949, and of Head of Household, 1951, England and Wales

Weekly Income of Chief Wage Earner[a]	Medical Consultation Rate[b]	
	Male	Female
1947		
Under £3	68	55
£3. to £5.10	38	38
£5.10 to £10	34	42
Over £10	39	49
Total	39	42
1949		
Under £3	89	63
£3 to £5 or £5.10	45	49
£5 or £5.10 to £10	34	44
Over £10	36	47
Total	41	49
1951		
Under £3	77	62
£3 to £5	59	56
£5 to £7.10	41	47
£7.10 to £10	36	44
Over £10	34	39
Total	47	51

Notes: a. In 1951, income group of head of household.
        b. The number of visits with a practitioner in a month per 100 persons interviewed.
Source: General Register Office, *The Survey of Sickness, 1943-52*, p. 57.

managerial and clerical occupations.[22] Over the period from 1947 to 1951, prevalence rates[23] for all males rose by 11 per cent while consultation rates rose by 20 per cent. The increase in consultation rates was greater than that in prevalence rates for men employed in professional and managerial occupations, manufacturing, mining and quarrying and building and roadmaking. Increases in consultation rates were lower than or close to changes in prevalence rates among clerical workers and men employed in distribution and agriculture.

What can we conclude from these data? Not, it seems, that lower income, working class patients were provided with considerably easier access to physician care after the introduction of the NHS. For one thing it is not immediately apparent that they made considerably less use of physician services than did middle class patients prior to 1948. Furthermore, among the section of the working class which most stood to benefit from the introduction of the new service — women — consultation rates did not increase to such an extent as among low income male patients. And the somewhat different images of the impact of the

NHS which are conveyed when analysing rates of consultation in relation to income and occupation, make it difficult to reach any firm conclusions as to the benefits working class patients derived from the service. It is true that the data leave much to be desired, but they do question the easy assumption that the NHS achieved a significant improvement in the access to care of working class patients.

Conclusion

In the process of planning the NHS, as well as in many of the earlier proposals for reform, the major emphasis was on the creation of a rational, efficent and nationally co-ordinated health service. Though not ignored, issues of class inequality were not a primary concern. But even so, we may ask what impact the service has had on the access to care of working class and middle class patients. The common view that socialised medicine is a response to the poor access of working class patients to care and to their demands for reform has often led to the easy assumption that they were the main beneficiaries of the NHS. But this ignores the fact that, for the first time, middle class patients were able to obtain care at no direct cost and were given access to the major hospitals, while still retaining the privilege of private medical care. Yet the initial impact of the service is difficult to assess, particularly its importance for working class patients. The limited data which are available on changes in consultation rates do not show consistent under-utilisation of health services on the part of working class patients before 1948, nor consistently greater increases in use of services than for middle class patients after the introduction of the new service. There is little to suggest that it was working class patients who benefited most from the new service and gained considerably easier access to care. But if we can reach no firm conclusions as to the immediate impact of the NHS on class patterns of use of services, perhaps we can more readily evaluate the operation of the service. The chapters which follow are concerned with the extent to which the NHS has provided equality of access to care and will examine class differences in access to general practitioner and hospital care. First, in order to provide a framework for this discussion, we will look at class variations in needs for care.

Notes

1. It was noted in the House of Commons that, in formulating plans for the reorganisation of the health services, Health Departments had been devoting particular attention to the proposals of the Medical Planning Commission and 'other professional views about the future of medical practice'. House of

7 CLASS DIFFERENCES IN NEEDS FOR HEALTH CARE

If equality of access to health care prevails, we would expect to find no differences in the quality of care received by patients of different social class, but we would not necessarily expect to find similar rates of use of services; equal rates of use do not signify equality of access if needs for health care are greater among working class than among middle class patients. In other words, data on different patterns of use of medical services are relatively meaningless if we have no indication of whether people's needs for professional diagnosis and treatment vary along social class lines or whether they are constant. Thus, any discussion of class differences in access to health care must be prefaced by an assessment of class variations in needs for care. Yet this is no simple task.[1]

In the first place, even if we have an adequate picture of the quality of health experienced in a given population, we can make no easy inferences as to the actual type or amount of medical services needed in that population. As anyone who is familiar with debates on the organisation and delivery of health care will know, the appropriateness of existing responses to illness is being questioned.[2] Have we, for example, too readily hospitalised patients when home based treatments would have been equally or more successful? Have patients developed an unhealthy dependence on doctors? Has the growth of individual and community responsibility for illness been stunted by too great a readiness on the part of the medical profession to define a wide range of problems as illnesses for which some form of professional action is appropriate? In such ways, automatic equations between illness and the need for medical care are being challenged and it is impossible to make any simple statements as to the amount or nature of health care necessary to treat a given level of illness in any population.

For the moment we can only look at broad differences in the quality of health of different classes and infer that higher levels of illness point to greater needs for care, without being able to specify more clearly the actual type or amount of services which are appropriate. But even when we seek to measure class variations in levels of health, we encounter problems. Due in part to a preoccupation with mortality data and, until recently, a relative neglect of morbidity patterns, existing measures of health are generally inadequate. In the compilation of health statistics, most emphasis has been placed upon vital statistics, particularly death rates. Health has traditionally been measured by the calculation of life expectancies, crude and age adjusted death rates and infant mortality. Despite some limitations, the reliability of these data is generally viewed as acceptable,[3] but they do not tell us enough about the quality of health of a population. The assumption is often made that improvements in mortality rates reflect improvements in health, yet the death rate tells us little about the living. While mortality rates for Britain have improved during the first half of this century, morbidity rates have been increasing — people with chronic illnesses who once would have died at a relatively early age are now having their lives prolonged by new drugs and treatments. But an index of health based on mortality rates alone shows us nothing of such changes in the incidence of chronic disease.

Given such changing patterns of disease, a greater emphasis is being placed upon the collection of morbidity statistics, yet the reliability and validity of these are also open to doubt. The most simple approach to the measurement of morbidity focuses on demands for medical care by compiling information on the rates of use of various health services. But need for care and use of services cannot be equated. Need stems from the incidence of illness while use of services reflects the interplay of illness and several other factors. Consequently, these data fail to capture those instances in which a need for care is not translated into a demand for such. They touch only the top of what Last has called a clinical 'iceberg' and his estimates suggest that a considerable amount of illness remains hidden.[4] Working on the basis of Last's estimates, Forsyth concludes that the population of England and Wales would contain

over two million with hypertensive heart disease, nearly half a million with urinary infections, three hundred thousand rheumatoid arthritics, an equal number of glycosurics, six hundred thousand bronchitics, and perhaps one and a half million people with conspicuous psychiatric disturbances. And none in receipt of medical treatment![5]

In an effort to obtain a more accurate image of the quality of health of people, various survey techniques have been developed. Some of these involve medical examinations of a sample population, while others focus on subjects' own reporting of symptoms and resulting disability.

to each other remained just about constant. A much more marked reduction occurred in post neo-natal death rates, yet here also, there was relatively little difference in the percentage decrease in rates for each of the classes. As with neo-natal mortality rates, class differences remained almost constant over the forty year period: in 1911 the rate for class V was almost 289 per cent higher than that for class I, and in 1949-50 it was just over 265 per cent higher.

These class inequalities have not been eradicated in more recent years. Statistics for 1964 indicate a continuation of these patterns — a further reduction in rates but no narrowing of class differences[8] — and census data for 1970-2, which are presented in Table 7.2, show more marked class inequalities, despite a general decrease in both neo-natal and post neo-natal death rates. We cannot make exact comparisons between 1949-50 and 1970-2 because of several classificatory changes, but it is worth noting that whereas the neo-natal death rate for class V

Table 7.2: Early Neo-natal, Late Neo-natal and Post Neo-natal Mortality Rates per 1,000 Live Births by Sex and Social Class, England and Wales, 1970-2

Social Class	Early neo-natal deaths[a]		Late neo-natal deaths[b]		Post neo-natal deaths[c]	
	males	females	males	females	males	females
I	8.89	6.31	1.23	0.99	3.47	2.32
II	9.73	7.43	1.39	1.29	4.09	3.22
III Non-manual	10.70	7.60	1.64	1.27	4.57	3.11
III Manual	11.04	8.27	1.81	1.53	6.20	4.99
IV	12.70	9.14	2.02	1.84	7.31	5.97
V	17.06	12.64	3.06	2.41	14.61	11.62
All classes	11.59	8.58	1.84	1.57	6.48	5.11
Per cent Excess V/I[d]	92	100	149	143	321	401

Notes: a. Deaths under 1 week
        b. Deaths between 1 and 3 weeks
        c. Deaths between 4 weeks and 1 year
        d. The difference between classes I and V expressed as a percentage of the rate for class I.

Source: Office of Population Censuses and Surveys, *Occupational Mortality. The Registrar General's Decennial Supplement for England and Wales 1970-72* (HMSO, London, 1978), p. 157.

in 1949-50 was 62 per cent higher than that for class I, in 1970-2 early and late neo-natal death rates for class V males and females were, with only one exception, over 100 per cent higher than for class I. Post neo-natal death rates followed the same pattern: whereas in 1949-50 the rate for class V was 265 per cent higher than for class I, in 1970-2 it was 321 per cent higher for males and 401 per cent higher for females.

The same pattern of consistently higher mortality rates for class V is also duplicated in rates for stillbirths and for maternal mortality. Stillbirths, presented in Table 7.3, follow a clear social class gradient and during the period from 1939 to 1970-2, the rates for class V increased

Table 7.3: Stillbirth Rates per 1,000 Single Births, Standardised for Mother's Age and Parity by Social Class, England and Wales, for Selected Years 1939-72

Social Class	1939	1949	Still births 1959-63	1970-72	
				males	females
I	23.4	14.3		8.63	8.92
II	29.3	18.9	12.8	10.16	10.01
III Non-manual	33.2	21.5	17.2	11.44	11.54
III Manual				12.26	12.81
IV	36.3	23.2	20.8	12.73	13.41
V	37.2	26.0		17.16	17.82
Per cent excess V/I[a]	59	82	63[b]	99	100

Notes: a.   The difference between classes I and V expressed as a percentage of the rate for class I.
   b.   Excess of rate for classes IV and V over that for classes I and II
Sources: J.N. Morris and J.A. Heady, 'Social and Biological Factors in Infant Mortality: V. Mortality in Relation to Father's Occupation, 1911-1950', *Lancet,* i (1955), p. 558; J.T. Hart, 'Data on Occupational Mortality 1959-63', *Lancet,* i (1972), p. 192; Office of Population Censuses and Surveys, *Occupational Mortality. The Registrar General's Decennial Supplement for England and Wales, 1970-72* (HMSO, London, 1978), p. 168.

from being 59 per cent higher than for class I to being almost 100 per cent higher. Also, the lower the social class of a woman, the more likely she is to die in childbirth. Standardised maternal mortality ratios have been consistently highest in lower social classes during the fifties, sixties and early seventies: while the ratios for class I women were 68 in 1949-53, 55 in 1962-5 and 79 in 1970-2, those for class V women were 132, 178 and 144 respectively.[9]

On the basis of such data on infant and maternal mortality, it is tempting to argue that there has been a gradual polarisation of the health experience of the classes, with the position of class V worsening relative to that of class I. This may indeed be so. But classificatory changes over the period we have surveyed make it impossible for us to argue this with any certainty. It is, however, quite obvious that mortality rates are consistently higher in lower social classes and, insofar

Commons, *Parliamentary Debates*, Fifth series, vol. 386 (HMSO, London, 1943), col. 1661.

2. Sir William Beveridge, *Report on Social Insurance and Allied Services* (HMSO, London,1942).

3. British Institute of Public Opinion, *The Beveridge Report and the Public* (British Institute of Public Opinion, London, n.d.).

4. House of Commons, *Parliamentary Debates*, vol. 386, col. 1661.

5. Ibid., col. 1664.

6. Ibid., vol. 397 (1944), col. 354-5.

7. Ibid., vol. 398 (1944), col. 428.

8. Ibid., vol. 422 (1946). For Bevan's speech to the House, see col. 43-63 and for the ensuing debate, col. 63-149, 200-313, 356-408.

9. It is not clear that the NHS was responsible for the redistribution of doctors. As Hart points out, the increased number of new doctors setting up in practice after the war had to take the only positions open to them — often in under-doctored areas. But the process of redistribution had stopped by 1956 and by 1961 it had reversed. Between 1961 and 1967 there was an increase from 17 per cent to 34 per cent in the proportion of people in under-doctored areas in England and Wales. Julian Tudor Hart, 'The Inverse Care Law', *Lancet*, i (1971), p. 408.

10. 'The National Health Service Act in Great Britain', *The Practitioner*, vol. 163 (1949).

11. Ibid., p. 96.

12. A. Lindsey, *Socialized Medicine in England and Wales* (University of North Carolina Press, Chapel Hill, NC, 1962), p. 72.

13. Data on hospital discharges in 1949 indicate that middle class patients fully availed themselves of this opportunity. These data are presented in Table 9.2. Brian Abel-Smith and Richard M. Titmuss, *The Cost of the National Health Service in England and Wales* (Cambridge University Press, Cambridge, 1956), p. 149.

14. Private hospital care is discussed in Ch. 9.

15. D. Mechanic, 'The English National Health Service: Some Comparisons with the United States', *Journal of Health and Social Behaviour*, vol. 12 (1971), p. 19.

16. It may well be the case that working class patients can less easily afford to pay for care during periods of unemployment and that they make less use of doctors than in periods of high employment.

17. D. Reid Ross, 'National Health Service in Factorytown: A Survey of the Demand for Medical Care in an Industrial Community', *Medical World*, vol. 78, no. 2 (1953), p. 129. As Ross points out, the community had been unusually prosperous since 1939 and this may have accounted for the apparent ease of access to medical care.

18. The *Survey of Sickness* provides data on morbidity and physician consultations for the period from 1943 to 1952 for a representative sample of the population aged 16 years and over. Unfortunately, the data for the earlier years are not always presented in relation to socio-economic variables.

19. Government Social Survey, *Survey of Sickness: October, 1943-December, 1945*, by P. Slater (HMSO, London, 1946), p. 72.

20. Class differences in needs for care are discussed more fully in Ch. 7.

21. This may reflect the difference between the sexes in the need to obtain medical legitimation in order to receive sickness cash benefits. Since most women were not paying health insurance, as they were not employed or else in part-time employment, they would not be entitled to a cash benefit while sick. The insured male would be.

22. General Register Office, *The Survey of Sickness, 1943-52*, Studies in

Medical and Population Subjects, no. 12 (HMSO, London, 1957), pp. 50-1.

23. The number of illnesses or injuries in a month per 100 persons interviewed.

as these rates can be taken as indices of needs for health care, they point to greater needs for care in classes IV and V.

Occupational Mortality

Occupational mortality data also suggest a growing disparity in the quality of health of different social classes. The most recent data are summarised in Table 7.4 in which standardised mortality ratios for men are presented by social class for four periods: 1930-2, 1949-53, 1959-63 and 1970-2. The occupations comprising each of the classes were modified in 1959-63 and so the 1949-53 rates are presented for both the old and new classifications. As before, such classificatory changes preclude detailed comparisons, but it seems that the benefits of the relative prosperity of the late fifties and sixties were not enjoyed by lower class males; the ratios for class V were markedly higher in 1959-63 and 1970-2 than in the earlier years. These inequalities in mortality rates among men are duplicated in the case of women, though class differences are less pronounced for single women than for married women. In 1949-53, the standardised mortality ratios for married women in classes I and V, were 96 and 110.[10] By 1970 these ratios were 89 and 156.[11]

Table 7.4: Standardised Mortality Ratios for Males by Social Class, England and Wales, for Selected Years 1930-72

Social Class	1930-2	1949-53	1949-53[a]	1959-63	1970-2
I	90	98	86	76	77
II	94	86	92	81	81
III	97	101	101	100	104
IV	102	94	104	103	114
V	111	118	118	143	137.

Note: a.   Adjusted to 1959-63 classification.
Sources: General Register Office, *The Registrar General's Decennial Supplement: England and Wales, 1961. Occupational Mortality. Tables* (HMSO, London, 1971), p. 22; Office of Population Censuses and Surveys, *Occupational Mortality. The Registrar General's Decennial Supplement for England and Wales, 1970-2* (HMSO, London, 1978), p. 174.

Mean annual death rates per 100,000 men by age and social class for 1930-2 and 1959-63 indicate an improvement in younger age groups for all social classes, though the reduction in rates is less marked for class V. This improvement continues in varying degree for older males in classes I, II and IV. For class III there is, however, an absolute increase over 1930-2 rates for men over 64, and in class V, for men over 55.[12] No allowance is made here for classificatory changes, but when the 1959-63 rates are adjusted for comparability, they are higher than the 1949-53 rates for men in class V; 102 per cent higher for those aged 55-64, 103 per cent higher for the 65-9 age group and 107 per cent higher for the 70-4 age group.[13] In fact, when 1961 and 1971 rates are adjusted according to the 1951 classification, there is minimal change in rates for class I and those for class V move from 118 in 1949-53, to 134 in 1959-63 and to 123 in 1970-2.[14] So while rates for men in each class at all ages have improved, the difference between classes I and V has widened and there has been an absolute increase in rates for certain age groups in class V. As a further example of the relative absence of change, it is interesting to note that in 1860-1 the death rate among miners of ages 45-54 was 115 per cent of that of all men at those ages while in 1959-63, the ratio was 112 per cent.[15]

This persistence of class differences in mortality rates is further illustrated when these rates are analysed by cause of death. Four diseases have traditionally been associated with poverty; respiratory tuberculosis, rheumatic heart disease, bronchitis and cancer of the stomach. Table 7.5 presents standardised mortality ratios for deaths from these and all causes for 1930-2, 1950 and 1970-2. Men in class V, compared with those in class I, have a far greater chance of dying of one of the four diseases and in each successive period there is an increasing difference in the health experience of the two classes. Except in the case of deaths from rheumatic heart disease, the differences in mortality ratios between classes I and V are greater in 1970-2 than in the earlier periods. Death rates from some other causes are, however, higher in social classes I and II: higher social classes are more prone to death from poliomyelitis, leukemia, cancer of the breast and cirrhosis of the liver.[16] But positive mortality gradients (where rates are high in low social classes) now extend to diabetes, vascular lesions of the nervous system, and coronary disease, and whereas there was no social class trend in deaths from lung cancer and duodenal ulcer in the mid 1930s, twenty years later mortality rates were highest in classes IV and V.[17]

These data suggest growing class inequalities. Class differences appear to have increased for infant mortality and for those diseases traditionally associated with poverty. At the same time, deaths from causes normally associated with class I are increasing in classes IV and V. For some diseases where once there were no class differences in mortality, rates are becoming proportionately higher for lower classes. At the moment we will simply note that these patterns exist and that they indicate that needs for health care are greater in classes IV and V. But

Table 7.5: Standardised Mortality Ratios for Deaths from Four Causes and All Causes for Adult Males Aged 20-64 Years[a] by Social Class, England and Wales 1930-2, 1950 and 1970-2

Cause of Death and Year	I	II	Social Class[b] III Non-manual	III Manual	IV	V
Respiratory t.b.:						
1930-2	61	70	100		104	125
1950	64	62	103		95	149
1970-2	26	41	84	89	124	254
Rheumatic heart disease:						
1930-2	65	92	97		111	112
1950	61	87	103		102	114
1970-2	77	80	117	103	116	124
Bronchitis:						
1930-2	31	57	91		124	146
1950	33	53	97		103	172
1970-2	36	51	82	113	128	188
Cancer of the stomach:						
1930-2	59	84	98		108	124
1950	57	67	100		114	132
1970-2	50	66	79	118	125	147
All causes:						
1930-2	90	94	97		102	111
1950	97	86	102		94	118
1970-2	77	81	99	106	114	137

Note: a. 15-64 years in 1970-2.

b. Class III, manual and non-manual combined in 1930-2 and 1950.

Sources: J.N. Morris and J.A. Heady, Social and Biological Factors in Infant Mortality: V. Mortality in Relation to Father's Occupation, 1911-1950, *Lancet*, i (1955), p. 557; Office of Population Censuses and Surveys, *Occupational Mortality. The Registrar General's Decennial Supplement for England and Wales. 1970-72* (HMSO, London, 1978), pp. 60-1.

we might also ask why these differences exist and consider their significance in assessing the success of the NHS (and social welfare legislation in general) in reducing class inequalities. We will return to these issues in the final chapter.

Class Differences in Morbidity

It is necessary to examine morbidity data also, in order to paint a more adequate picture of class differences in health. But since a certain amount of illness will never be seen by doctors, it is unwise to rely on data based on treatments received from doctors and hospitals, for this will lead to an underestimation of morbidity. It is more useful therefore, to concentrate on survey data which will include illnesses never presented to doctors. Unfortunately there are relatively few such sources of data for Britain which are analysed in terms of social class — an indication, perhaps, of the relative complacency about the extent to which the NHS meets the needs of different classes.

There are, however, two major sources of morbidity data which are useful; the *Survey of Sickness* which started in 1943 and continued until 1952, and the *Government Household Survey* which is published annually. In the *Survey of Sickness* a person was considered to be ill if he or she felt ill, but different dimensions of illness were conveyed through three different measures; the sickness rate was defined as the percentage of people reporting some illness or injury in a month; the prevalence rate was defined as the number of illnesses or injuries per 100 persons in a month (this can exceed 100); and the incapacity rate indicates the number of days off work or confined to the house in a month per 100 persons interviewed. The data for January 1946 indicate no clear pattern in the morbidity experience of different occupational groups — the two highest status groups do not have sickness, prevalence or incapacity rates which are consistently lower than the blue-collar groups. The highest sickness rates are experienced by the mining and quarrying group, and the retired and unoccupied — the particularly high rate for the former being reflected in the high incapacity rate for this group. But it is the retired and unoccupied who have the highest prevalence rate, suggesting that sickness is a more pervasive feature of life for these people.[18]

Data for the remaining years of the survey are more suggestive of a relationship between social class and morbidity, though differences which exist between high and low income groups become less marked when the data are analysed by occupation. For example, during 1947, 1949, and 1951, persons in lower income groups had higher sickness, prevalence and incapacity rates than those in higher income groups,[19] but there were no marked differences in sickness and prevalence rates for different occupational groups.[20] Yet one persistent difference remains in an occupational analysis; incapacity rates are generally lower for non-manual workers than for those in manual occupations and in the retired and unoccupied category. From July 1947 to June 1949, for example, incapacity rates were nearly 40 per cent higher for manual workers than for those in non-manual occupations.[21] Jewkes argues that absences from work are more frequent where sick benefits and/or wages are paid during periods of disability, and that they tend to increase with the generosity of sickness payments.[22] But this observation cannot be used to explain the higher incapacity rates of lower class workers. It is these workers who are most likely to experience severe financial problems as a result of disability[23] and absence from work has been shown to be independent of the availability of sick pay schemes.[24] For lower status occupational groups and for the retired and unoccupied, illness appears to be of greater severity and longer duration than for those of higher occupational status.

This same image of a greater amount of ill health among working class people is also conveyed by the *General Household Survey*. In most of the years for which the survey has reported there is a clear inverse relationship between socio-economic status and prevalence of chronic and acute illness. The data for 1974, which are presented in Table 7.6, follow a similar pattern to those for other years. As socio-economic status declines there is for both men and women, an increase in chronic illness, in the proportion of respondents reporting restricted activity and in the average number of days of restricted activity experienced during the course of the year. The rate for long standing illness for men in the unskilled manual group is 118 per cent higher than for men in professional occupations and for women the rate is 104 per cent higher. For limiting long standing illness the rates were 174 per cent and 146 per cent higher respectively. Compared with men and women in the professional group, 50 per cent more men in unskilled manual work and 22 per cent of the women reported restricted activity and on average they experienced 115 per cent and 51 per cent more days of restricted activity. Only in 1975 does this pattern change slightly; instead of a continuous social class gradient in the reporting of acute illness, the rates rise with declining socio-economic status but then fall off slightly for the unskilled manual group.[25]

In addition to these two major surveys, there are a number of more limited studies which provide us with information on the morbidity experienced by different social classes and which generally confirm this picture of greater morbidity in lower social classes. A Political and Economic Planning survey in mid-1957 in Northampton and the Greater London area asked a random sample of mothers whether they thought their health was good. The percentages who believed their health was *not* too good increased with decreasing occupational status; 11 per cent of those in the managerial and professional category; 14 per cent in the supervisory, technical and clerical personnel category; 17 per cent in the skilled worker, and 27 per cent in the unskilled worker cate-

Table 7.6: Chronic and Acute Illness Rates by Socio-economic Group and Sex, Great Britain, 1974

	Socio-economic Group						
	Professional	Employers and Managers	Intermediate and Junior Non-manual	Skilled Manual	Semi-skilled Manual	Unskilled Manual	All
Men							
Chronic illness:							
Long standing illness[a]	141	185	226	202	222	308	206
Limiting long standing illness[a]	82	113	147	132	147	225	134
Acute illness:							
Restricted activity in two week period[a]	74	83	99	96	99	111	93
Average number of days of restricted activity per person per year	10.8	14.2	14.5	18.6	18.3	23.2	16.8
Women							
Chronic illness:							
Long standing illness[a]	154	176	222	198	280	314	224
Limiting long standing illness[a]	93	115	143	124	198	229	150
Acute illness:							
Restricted activity in two week period[a]	94	88	104	96	108	115	99
Average number of days of restricted activity per person per year	14.2	17.0	18.4	17.5	20.5	21.4	18.3

Note: a.   Rates per 1,000.
Source: Office of Population Censuses and Surveys, Social Survey Division, *The General Household Survey 1974* (HMSO, London, 1977), pp. 155, 157, 160.

gories.[26] The College of General Practitioners' study of the incidence of chronic bronchitis among men and women aged 45-64 years revealed a greater incidence of bronchitis among lower class persons, the difference being only partly explained by differences in smoking habits. Even when more rigid criteria of classifying bronchitics were used, the social class gradient was still obvious.[27] Dunnell and Cartwright note a positive social class gradient in the number of symptoms which subjects reported and in the proportion who rated their health as fair or poor,[28] and two surveys which provide us with information on childhood morbidity indicate a rise in the incidence of infective illness from classes I to V in the first two years of life.[29]

Conclusion

Mortality and morbidity data consistently point to a greater experience of ill health among working class patients and thus needs for health care appear to increase as social class declines. I have already pointed to some of the problems inherent in these data, but it is worth reiterating that a proportion of the symptoms which are experienced by people, whether or not they result in disability, are not such as to require professional diagnosis and treatment. The reporting of illness and incapacity cannot necessarily be equated with a need for medical care. However, in the absence of more sophisticated measures, we have to rely on the clues provided by existing morbidity and mortality data, and if equality of access to care prevails within the NHS, these lead us to expect higher rates of consultation on the part of working class patients. While I will not dwell on the issue at the moment, it is important to note that, in addition to providing a framework for a discussion of the extent to which the NHS provides equal access to care, these unchanging patterns of mortality and morbidity are also an indictment of the NHS. Quite obviously, the NHS, and social welfare legislation in general, have proved to be remarkably ineffective in reducing class inequalities in health.

Notes

1, For a discussion of methodological problems in developing indices of health, see US Department of Health, Education and Welfare, Public Health Service, National Centre for Health Statistics, *Conceptual Problems in Developing an Index of Health*, Vital and Health Statistics, series 2, no. 17 (Government Printing Office, Washington, DC, 1966).

2. See, for example, Ivan Illich, *Limits to Medicine* (McClelland and Stewart, Toronto, 1976).

3. The reliability and validity of mortality and morbidity data are discussed in Paul W. Haberman, 'The Reliability and Validity of the Data' in J. Kosa *et al.* (eds.), *Poverty and Health* (Harvard University Press, Cambridge, Mass., 1969).

4. J.M. Last 'The Iceberg: Completing the Picture in General Practice', *Lancet*, ii (1963), pp. 28-31.

5. Gordon Forsyth, *Doctors and State Medicine: A Study of the British Health Service* (Pitman Medical Publishing Co. Ltd, London, 1966), pp. 63-4.

6. US Department of Health Education and Welfare, p. 14.

7. The data on class differences in health and access to care are frequently classified in terms of the Registrar General's classification. This is largely based on occupation, but it also takes into account 'standing within the community', and the correlation of occupational position with similarities of 'social, cultural and recreational standards and behaviour'. In general, class I may be seen as comprising higher professional and managerial occupations; class II, lower profes-

sional; class III, clerical and skilled manual occupations; class IV, semi-skilled manual occupations and class V, unskilled manual occupations.

8. There was a 38 per cent decrease in neo-natal death rates for classes I and II and a 30 per cent decrease for class IV and V between 1949 and 1964. For post neo-natal rates, there was a 52 per cent decrease for classes I and II and a 56 per cent decrease for classes IV and V. General Register Office, *Regional and Social Factors in Infant Mortality*, by C.C. Spicer and L. Lipworth, Studies in Medical and Population Subjects, no. 19 (HMSO, London, 1966), p. 15.

9. General Register Office, *The Registrar General's Decennial Supplement: England and Wales, 1951. Occupational Mortality*, Part II, vol. 2 (HMSO, London, 1957), p. 346; ibid., *The Registrar General's Decennial Supplement: England and Wales, 1961. Occupational Mortality* (HMSO, London, 1971), p. 503; Office of Population Censuses and Surveys, *Occupational Mortality. The Registrar General's Decennial Supplement for England and Wales, 1970-72* (HMSO, London, 1978), p. 156. No adjustment is made for classificatory changes.

10. General Register Office, *The Registrar General's Decennial Supplement: England and Wales 1951*, p. 2.

11. Office of Population Censuses and Surveys, *Occupational Mortality*, p. 217.

12. General Register Office, *The Registrar General's Decennial Supplement: England and Wales, 1961*, p. 28.

13. Ibid., p. 24.

14. Office of Population Censuses and Surveys, *Occupational Mortality*, p. 174.

15. General Register Office, *The Registrar General's Decennial Supplement: England and Wales, 1961*, p. 1.

16. M.W. Susser and W. Watson, *Sociology in Medicine*, 2nd edn (Oxford University Press, London 1971), Ch. 4.

17. General Register Office, *The Registrar General's Decennial Supplement: England and Wales, 1961*; 'Health and Social Class', *Lancet*, i (1959), pp. 303-5.

18. Government Social Survey, *Survey of Sickness: October, 1943-December 1945*, by P. Slater (HMSO, London, 1946), p. 72.

19. Ibid., p. 57.

20. Ibid., pp. 50-1.

21. W.P.D. Logan, 'Illness, Incapacity and Medical Attention Among Adults, 1947-49', *Lancet*, i (1950), p. 775.

22. J. Jewkes and S. Jewkes, *Value for Money in Medicine* (Basil Blackwell, Oxford, 1963).

23. It may be that people in higher status occupations are more motivated to return earlier to their work (which is often more congenial) and that they are, therefore, incapacitated for shorter periods of time. But the financial problems of workers in lower status occupations may counteract this effect. Ann Cartwright, *Patients and Their Doctors: A Study of General Practice* (Routledge and Kegan Paul, London, 1967).

24. Office of Population Censuses and Surveys, Social Survey Division, *The General Household Survey* (HMSO, London, 1973), p. 308.

25. Ibid. (1978), p. 145.

26. Politcal and Economic Planning, *Family Needs and the Social Services* (Allen and Unwin, London, 1961), p. 82.

27. College of General Practitioners, 'Chronic Bronchitis in Great Britain', *British Medical Journal*, vol. 2 (1961), pp. 973-9.

28. Karen Dunnell and Ann Cartwright, *Medicine Takers, Prescribers and Hoarders* (Routledge and Kegan Paul, London, 1972), p. 51.

29. J.W.B. Douglas and J.M. Blomfield, *Children Under Five* (Allen and Unwin, London, 1958); J. Spence, *et al.*, *A Thouand Families in Newcastle-Upon-Tyne* (Oxford University Press, London, 1954); F.J.W. Miller *et al.*, *Growing Up in Newcastle-Upon-Tyne* (Oxford University Press, London, 1960).

8 CLASS DIFFERENCES IN ACCESS TO GENERAL PRACTITIONER CARE

The general practitioner is the cornerstone of the NHS; he or she provides first contact care and, where necessary, refers patients to specialists or admits them to hospital. Consultations with specialists can only be obtained by referral from a GP. Access to care from general practitioners is, therefore, crucial in that this is the patient's main entry point to the health care system.[1] Unfortunately few studies have sought to determine whether patients of different social class receive care of the same quality and whether their use of GP services reflects their needs for care. A general belief that the NHS was among the most successful of the post-war reforms seems to have inhibited research on many aspects of the service. Moreover, those studies which have been concerned with class variations in consultation rates have pointed to different conclusions and have provoked some debate as to whether working class patients are disadvantaged in their access to care.[2] Any assessment of the NHS will depend on the information which is available to us and the kinds of measures which are used to assess the effectiveness of the services. With respect to class inequalities in access to care, the data which are available leave much to be desired and it is difficult to appreciate their significance. Bearing this in mind, let us look at those studies which provide us with information on class patterns of consultation with general practitioners.

Rates of Use of General Practitioner Services

Several studies lead us to suppose that working class patients make less use of GP services than we would expect on the basis of their needs for care. The General Register Office survey of general practice which covered the period from May 1955 to April 1956 provides us with information from 76 practices in England and Wales. Patient consulting rates for children and for adult males in this study are shown in Table 8.1. The patient consulting rate refers to the number of persons per 1,000 who had one or more consultations with a GP during the study period. Thus it tells us something about the proportion of patients in each class who received treatment, but nothing of the frequency with which doctors were consulted by these patients. The study gives us no valid estimate of the needs for care within the

Table 8.1: Patient Consulting Rates for Children Under 15 Years and Males Aged 15-64 Years by Social Class with Occupational Breakdowns for Classes III, IV and V, May 1955-April 1956

Social Class	Patient Consulting Rates[a]			
	Children		Adult Males	
I Professional, managerial	671		544	
II Intermediate	680		557	
III Skilled:	720		602	
(a) Mineworkers		707		721
(b) Transport workers		712		591
(c) Clerical workers		727		575
(d) Others		722		603
IV Partly skilled:	679		578	
(a) Agricultural workers		591		452
(b) Others		723		653
V Unskilled:	667		579	
(a) Building and dock labourers		695		577
(b) Others		654		580
All classes	699		585	

Note: a.   The number of patients per 1,000 who had one or more consultations during the twelve months.

Source: General Register Office, *Morbidity Statistics from General Practice*, by W.P.D. Logan and A.A. Cushion, Studies in Medical and Population Subjects, II, no. 14 (HMSO, London, 1960), pp. 78, 151.

population studied, but viewed in the light of national patterns of mortality and morbidity, these rates suggest an underutilisation of general practitioners on the part of some working class patients. We would expect the rates to rise through classes I to V, but in the case of both children and adult males there is a fall in rates for classes IV and V. In fact, the rates for class V and for agricultural workers in class IV are below the average for all classes.

This image of inequality is also confirmed by other studies. In Cartwright's survey of general practice, she notes that, at first, there appeared to be an inverse relationship between social class and consultation rates, but that when the data were analysed by age, many of the differences disappeared.[3] Among those under 45 years of age, the working class patients had higher consultation rates than the middle class — 53 per cent higher. But there was little difference between working and middle class patients aged 45-74 years, and among the patients aged 75 years and over, the middle class were more likely to consult their doctor than the working class. Thus, guided by national patterns of morbidity and mortality — for Cartwright does not provide us with any index of the health needs of the middle class and working class patients in her sample — it would seem that working class patients over 45 years of age were at a disadvantage in their access to general practitioner care. In another study in which she collaborated with Dunnell, class differences in consultation rates paralleled variations in morbidity, but these data are not presented in relation to age.[4]

Other studies, concerned with particular areas in England provide us with additional information and these also suggest that working class patients may underutilise GP services. For, given our expectation of higher rates of use on the part of class IV and class V patients, then equal rates of consultation or just small differences in rates between working class and middle class patients lead us to conclude an inequality in access to care. Kedward's study of a general practice in Nottinghamshire indicates that a higher proportion of blue collar households consulted a doctor during the survey period, but there were only small class differences in the average number of consultations.[5] Kessel and Shepherd examined the attendance patterns of the 1,503 people who were continuously registered with a practice in Beckenham during the first ten years of the NHS.[6] They classified these patients as either 'attenders' or 'non-attenders'; attenders had consulted a doctor in 1957 or 1958 while non-attenders had last consulted a doctor in 1956 or earlier. They found no class differences between these categories, and the non-attenders appeared to be healthy. Stein's study of a London general practice found that the percentage of attenders and the mean number of consultations was higher in classes IV and V, but the differences between the classes were not statistically significant.[7] Also, a study by Ashford and Pearson of NHS patients registered with general practitioners in Exeter, shows a tendency for the number of patient contacts to increase slightly with decreasing social class and decreasing educational level.[8] But the charts which the authors present indicate less clear 'general tendencies' than they suggest in their text.

In none of these studies is there evidence that class patterns of consultation parallel the needs for care of working class and middle class patients. Rather, they raise the possibility that working class patients underutilise GP services. But these studies are difficult to interpret for they provide us with no indication of patients' needs for care and we can only be guided by national patterns of mortality and morbidity. One early study which does provide us with both rates of consultation and measures of morbidity (in the form of sickness, prevalence and incapacity rates) is the *Survey of Sickness*. As can be seen in Table 8.2, the rates of consultation in 1949 and 1951 for different income categories generally paralleled the morbidity of these groups; sickness, prevalence and incapacity rates are highest for low income groups and so also are consultation rates. But, depending on which measure of morbidity we take as the most valid index of needs for health care, we are led to different conclusions. When consultation rates are matched against incapacity rates, there is evidence that lower income patients underutilise GP services. In 1949, the incapacity rate for men in the lower income group was 295 per cent higher than in the highest income group, while the consultation rate was only 147 per cent higher. This same pattern can be seen in the data for 1951 although the differences are less pronounced. The comparable figures for women were 87 per cent and 34 per cent in 1949, though in 1951, variations in consultation rates paralleled those in incapacity rates. If, on the other hand, we take prevalence rates as the most valid index of morbidity — and this does seem reasonable, as it is this which indicates the episodes of illnesses and injuries — then consultation rates for both years suggest equality of access, or even an underutilisation of physicians by middle class patients. In 1949, for example, the prevalence rates for the lowest income group were 80 per cent higher for men and 35 per cent higher for women than those for the top income group; consultation rates were 147 per cent and 34 per cent higher, respectively.

In the face of such contradictory patterns we are simply left with questions. Can we apply national patterns of morbidity and mortality to the smaller scale studies of class differences in consultations with GPs? What are the most useful measures of needs for care? Is it indeed reasonable to focus on prevalence rates? Do the differences between the studies reflect such methodological problems or are they a reflection of changing patterns of use? Is it the case that in the early years of the NHS there was a relative equality of access which then diminished during the fifties and sixties?

The most recent information on patterns of consultation with general practitioners is that which is published annually in the *General Household Survey*; this also provides us with morbidity data. The pattern which emerges is somewhat different than in the *Survey of Sickness,* though hardly less confusing. If, for 1974, we compare one measure of acute illness — the rate per 1,000 people reporting restricted activity in a two week period — with the rate per 1,000 people consulting a GP in the same period, then we find some correspondence between differences in morbidity and in the use of GP services by different socioeconomic groups. For example, for men in unskilled manual work, the restricted activity rate was 50 per cent higher than for men in professional occupations, while the consultation rate was 41 per cent

Table 8.2: Mean Monthly Sickness, Prevalence, Incapacity and Medical Consultation Rates per 100 Persons Interviewed by Sex and Weekly Income, England and Wales, 1949 and 1951.

	Sickness rate[a]		Prevalence rate[b]		Incapacity rate[c]		Medical Consultation rate[d]	
	Men	Women	Men	Women	Men	Women	Men	Women
Income Group of Chief Wage-earner	**1949**							
Under £3	82	83	198	214	261	159	89	63
£3 and under £5 or £5.10	63	74	121	169	113	111	45	49
£5 or £5.10 and under £10	61	73	112	161	84	92	34	44
£10 and over	59	71	110	158	66	85	36	47
Not known	59	73	109	164	69	94	33	48
Total	63	74	121	171	104	107	41	49
% excess lowest/highest income group[e]	39	17	80	35	295	87	147	34
Income Group of Head of Household	**1951**							
Under £3	77	82	171	202	198	139	77	62
£3 and under £5	71	76	151	176	179	133	59	56
£5 and under £7.10	65	73	119	162	112	100	41	47
£7.10 and under £10	63	71	112	153	76	97	36	44
£10 and over	63	71	113	145	72	91	34	39
Not known	62	72	111	156	92	97	45	46
Total	67	75	127	170	119	111	47	51
% excess lowest/highest income group[e]	22	15	51	39	175	53	126	59

Note: a.   Number of people per 100 reporting some illness or injury in a month.
        b.   Number of illnesses or injuries in a month per 100 people interviewed.
        c.   Number of days off work or confined to the house in a month per 100 people interviewed.
        d.   Number of visits in a month to or by a medical practitioner per 100 people interviewed. (This includes general practitioners and medically qualified ophthalmic and other specialists but excludes dentists and care received while a hospital in-patient)
        e.   Calculated from the rates in the table. The difference between the highest and lowest income groups expressed as a percentage of the rate for the highest income group.

Source: General Register Office, *The Survey of Sickness 1943 to 1952*, by W.P.D. Logan and E.M. Brooke, Studies in Medical and Population Subjects, no. 12 (HMSO, London, 1957), p. 57.

higher and the average number of consultations was 46 per cent higher. For women from the same socio-economic groups, the restricted activity rate was 22 per cent higher, the consultation rate 23 per cent higher and the average number of consultations 18 per cent higher for the unskilled manual group.[9] But in the case of the other indices of morbidity (measures of chronic illness and days of restricted activity) the differences between the socio-economic groups were much greater. Were we to rely on these, we would be led to the conclusion that there is a considerable inequality in the access which these groups have to general practitioners.[10]

This evidence of inequality can also be seen in the data from the *General Household Survey* for 1975. As Table 8.3 shows, when measures of chronic illness are compared with consultation rates, then it appears that patients of lower socio-economic status underutilised GP services. For example, the long-standing illness rate for men in the unskilled manual group was 97 per cent higher than that for men in the professional group, but the consultation rate was only 11 per cent higher. The difference was even greater for women in these groups. But the pattern of acute illness is somewhat different than in 1974 and does not show quite the same correspondence with consultation rates as in the previous year. In neither of the measures of acute illness is there a smooth social class gradient and although consultation rates tend to parallel these variations, they are relatively low for the semi-skilled and unskilled manual groups. Moreover, when these rates are broken down by age, there is some evidence that men and women aged 15-44 in lower socio-economic groups are at a disadvantage in access to GP care[11] — the age group which, in Cartwright's study, seemed to enjoy equal access to doctors.[12] The patterns within the *General Household Survey* data are somewhat difficult to identify and it would certainly be an aid in understanding the significance of the data if information on rates of consultation were standardised in terms of various measures of need. To what extent are the consultations a response to either acute or chronic illness and how many serve an administrative function, providing a sickness certificate or a repeat of a prescription and nothing else? Are the people who report illness, the ones who are consulting a physician? It would be useful to have answers to such questions.

On the basis of these various studies, it is difficult to judge whether working class patients enjoy equal access to care. Some evidence points in this direction. But other data suggest that, compared with middle class patients, working class patients may consult general practitioners less frequently than morbidity and mortality rates would lead us to expect. Some studies have focused on preventive care and indicate class

Table 8.3: Chronic and Acute Illness and Consultation Rates by Socio-economic Group and Sex, Great Britain, 1975

Socio-economic Group	Chronic Illness		Acute Illness		Consultations	
	Long standing illness[a]	Limiting long standing illness[b]	Restricted activity[c]	Average number of days of restricted activity[d]	Consultation rate[e]	Average number of consultations[f]
MEN						
1. Professional	168	93	91	13.5	85	2.7
2. Employers and managers	216	131	75	12.9	83	2.7
3. Intermediate and junior non-manual	229	150	87	14.9	96	3.1
4. Skilled manual	227	143	90	16.1	95	3.0
5. Semi-skilled manual	268	162	93	17.6	104	3.5
6. Unskilled manual	331	227	77	16.3	94	3.3
All	231	144	86	15.3	93	3.0
% excess 6/1[g]	97	144	-15	21	11	22
WOMEN						
1. Professional	149	76	83	16.2	114	3.5
2. Employers and managers	212	124	87	15.7	119	3.5
3. Intermediate and junior non-manual	244	152	99	17.3	126	4.2
4. Skilled manual	216	139	95	16.4	115	3.6
5. Semi-skilled manual	293	197	111	22.1	135	4.3
6. Unskilled manual	377	263	106	20.9	126	3.8
All	246	159	98	17.9	122	3.0
% excess 6/1[g]	153	246	28	29	11	9

Notes:
a. Persons aged 15 years and over reporting long standing illness, per 1,000.
b. Persons aged 15 years and over reporting limiting long standing illness, per 1,000.
c. Rates per 1,000 reporting restricted activity in a two week reference period.
d. Average number of restricted activity days per person per year.
e. Persons consulting a general practitioner (NHS) in a two week reference period, rates per 1,000.
f. Average number of general practitioner (NHS) consultations per person per year.
g. Calculated from rates in the table. The difference between Group 1 and Group 6 expressed as a percentage of the rate for Group 1.

Source: Office of Population Censuses and Surveys, Social Survey Division, *The General Household Survey, 1975* (HMSO, London, 1978), pp. 140, 142, 145, 149.

differences in the use of these services also. A study published by the Government Social Survey in 1952 shows that the groups of mothers who were least co-operative in having their children immunised were less well educated, from poorer households, and had several children. Few of these mothers had their children immunised and an even smaller proportion had them immunised at the right age. They were also unlikely to have had their children vaccinated against smallpox.[13] A clinic for cervical cytology in Derby was attended mainly by women belonging to classes I and II and the upper part of class III and only with the introduction of a domiciliary service, with most cases chosen by health visitors on social grounds, was the class balance redressed.[14] Similarly, a health screening clinic in Rotherham was visited mainly by people of middle class background.[15]

Whether family planning advice can be equated with other types of preventive care is not clear, but a study by Cartwright has shown class variations in methods of contraception and in the sources of advice on birth control which are consulted.[16] This was a survey in twelve registration districts in England and Wales and the sample covered mothers and some fathers of babies aged between four and nine months. There were no social class differences in the number of children mothers hoped for when they married, but working class mothers had more unintentional pregnancies. They were less likely to use a method of birth control and were also less likely than middle class mothers to use effective methods of contraception. The proportion of mothers seeking professional advice on birth control rose with the number of children they had, but mothers with husbands in non-manual jobs were more likely to have discussed family planning with professionals than were mothers with husbands in manual jobs (even though the latter had more children). This trend was especially marked for Family Planning Clinics and somewhat less so for GPs, although discussions with health visitors were more frequent for working class mothers.[17]

In the absence of more information and more sophisticated measures which relate utilisation of services to need, it is difficult to add to the debate over the extent to which the NHS provides equal access to care for patients of different social class. There is supportive evidence for those on each side of the debate. In the case of two measures of morbidity — prevalence rates in the *Survey of Sickness* and people reporting restricted activity in the *General Household Survey* — there is a rough correspondence with class differences in consultation rates. But no single index of needs for health care is adequate in itself, and in the case of other measures of morbidity and mortality, class differences are not matched by variations in consultation rates. While the picture is not as clear as we might wish, this evidence of inequality does mean that complacency should be abandoned in favour of critical research. There is a need for the development of more valid and reliable measures of utilisation in relation to needs for care. Also, our understanding of data on rates of consultation would be enhanced by studies which more thoroughly explore class differences in responses to symptoms of illness — how symptoms are perceived, what action is taken to cope with them, when and why professional advice is sought and to what extent patients are satisfied with the advice and treatment they receive. But access to care is not only measured by rates of use of services, it is also important to look at the quality of care which patients of different social class receive. It is possible, for example, that inequalities in the use of GP services are compounded by differences in the quality of care received by patients, which are such as to place middle class patients in an even more advantageous position.

Variations in Quality of Care

The few studies which have focused on class variations in quality of care suggest that working class patients may be receiving care of lesser quality. In a study of a representative sample of people who had been hospitalised sometime during the six months before the survey period, Cartwright obtained data on the care they received from general practitioners.[18] The results suggest that middle class patients may obtain a rather better service from their general practitioners; doctors practicing in middle class areas had smaller lists; a higher proportion had further qualifications; more had graduated from Oxford, Cambridge, or London; twice as many had a hospital appointment or hospital beds; and a higher proportion had direct access to X-ray equipment and physiotherapy.[19] Fourteen per cent of middle class patients were visited by their general practitioner in hospital while only four per cent of working class patients received such a visit, and there was evidence that doctors were more likely to send their middle class patients directly to hospital. In her later study of general practice, Cartwright sought confirmation of these differences, yet she found no significant variations between middle class and working class patients in the size of their doctor's list, though those in professional occupations were rather more likely to be on small lists of under 2,000.[20] Patients in the professions were also most likely to have doctors who had qualified since 1945, and middle class patients were more likely to have doctors with hospital appointments. But there were no differences in the proportion of doc-

tors who had access to hospital beds or other facilities; in the number
of procedures carried out by doctors in their own practices; in the
membership of doctors in the College of General Practitioners; in their
views on preventive care and in their enjoyment of general practice.[21]
On the basis of these results, Cartwright modifies her original hypo-
thesis and suggests that only patients in the professions seem to get
better care.

Whereas Cartwright uses several different indices to assess variations
in quality of care, Taylor's comments on the standard of work of
general practitioners are much more impressionistic.[22] In a study which
was largely an effort to brighten the dismal picture of general practice
painted by Collings,[23] Taylor interviewed and observed at work ninety-
four general practitioners who were recognised by their colleagues as
good doctors. The explicit purpose of the study was to describe the
best in the general practitioner service. It was in the working class
industrial areas that he found the poorer practices. Doctors in these
areas tended to have the largest lists of patients while those in middle
class urban-residential areas generally had smaller lists. Most doctors
were providing their patients with a high standard of care, but the
working class areas did contain a substantial minority 'who fail to give
their patients the service they have a right to expect'.[24] The doctors
working in these areas did so for a variety of reasons. For some, there
was no other choice; they lacked the ability to work in better areas. For
others, there was a financial incentive, their aim being to make as much
money as possible in a short period and then leave the area. These,
Taylor argues, were giving their patients no more than a good garage
mechanic offers to his customers. There were also those who worked
in such areas from a sense of vocation, but many of these would bow
under the strain of a heavy work load and become mediocre doctors.
It was among the doctors in these areas that low morale was most
common:

> It is here that the potentially good general practitioner will most
> often complain of frustration; the less conscientious general practi-
> tioner will undergo a lowering of standards, without himself realizing
> what has happened; lack of contact with colleagues is most marked;
> and the need to raise the standards of general practice is most
> obvious.[25]

Given the aim of Taylor — to show the best in the general practitioner
service —we may perhaps place more reliance on his negative observa-

tions than if his aim had been quite the opposite.

The quality of care which a patient obtains will not only depend on the doctor he consults, for the patient can play a role in determining the care that he or she receives. The nature of the doctor-patient relationship appears to vary according to whether patients are working class or middle class. Rates of consultation may, therefore, be an inadequate measure of the extent to which patients receive care commensurate with their needs, because middle class patients may be able to obtain more from any single consultation. They are, for example, more likely to play an active part in the doctor-patient relationship while working class patients are more passive. Titmuss has argued that the working class patient is more easily disciplined and managed and he expressed the hope that a generally higher standard of education would 'herald the gradual disappearance of an uncomplaining, subservient, class-saturated acceptance of low standards of professional service'.[26] Also, Collings noted that middle class patients tended to be resented by general practitioners because of their demands for more time and attention, and a readiness to question diagnoses, to seek reasons for statements and instructions, and even to challenge the doctor. Their 'less fortunate neighbours' were more respectful of their doctors' expert knowledge and skills.[27] Similarly, Cartwright indicates that the higher a patient's social class position, the longer the consultation is likely to last and the more likely it is that the patient will discuss several problems with the doctor and ask for information about his illness and its treatment.[28] And Taylor observed that

> the doctors in the industrial areas tend to have specially friendly and uncritical relations with their patients, each taking the other side as it finds it. Indeed, those doctors with mixed urban-residential and industrial practices almost always prefer their working class patients, because they are less exacting and more appreciative.[29]

There appear to be few other studies which are concerned with the quality of care received by patients of different social class. Once again, we are faced with a paucity of data. Yet, given the inequalities which these studies suggest, there seems to be little foundation for the general complacency about the success of the NHS in meeting the needs for care of working class and middle class patients.

Conclusion

A variety of studies indicate class inequalities in access to care under the

NHS. Working class patients consult with GPs less frequently than we would expect on the basis of certain measures of morbidity and there is evidence that the care which they receive is of lesser quality than that received by middle class patients. But what is most striking, is that so few studies have questioned whether working class patients are disadvantaged in their access to care. The assumption that the NHS was directed at removing class inequalities in access to care has been matched by a remarkable complacency. It is true that there are many problems in developing reliable and valid indices of needs for care and the quality of care provided by doctors. But there appear to have been few attempts to surmount these problems. The data which are available leave much to be desired and do not point consistently to the conclusion that working class patients have less access to care than do their middle class counterparts. Yet this is a sufficiently common pattern, that we need to abandon the complacency of past years and more closely examine the issue of class inequalities in access to care.

Notes

1. In this and the following chapter, access to care refers to rates of use of medical services by different social classes and also variations in the quality of care received.

2. Rein and Mechanic have both argued that the NHS provides equal access to health care. M. Rein, 'Social Class and the Utilization of Medical Care Services', *Hospitals*, vol. 43 (1 July 1969), pp. 43-54; D. Mechanic, 'The English National Health Service: Some Comparisons With the United States', *Journal of Health and Social Behaviour*, vol. 12 (1971), pp. 18-29. For an argument to the contrary, see Julian Tudor Hart, 'The Inverse Care Law', *Lancet*, i (1971), pp. 405-12.

3. Ann Cartwright, *Patients and Their Doctors: A Study of General Practice* (Routledge and Kegan Paul, London, 1967).

4. Karen Dunnell and Ann Cartwright, *Medicine Takers, Prescribers and Hoarders* (Routledge and Kegan Paul, London, 1972).

5. H.B. Kedward, 'Social Class Habits of Consulting',*British Journal of Preventive and Social Medicine*, vol. 16, no. 3 (1962), pp. 147-52.

6. N. Kessel and M. Shepherd, 'The Health and Attitudes of People Who Seldom Consult a Doctor', *Medical Care*, vol. 3, no. 1 (1965), pp. 6-10.

7. L. Stein, 'Morbidity in a London General Practice: Social and Demographic Data', *British Journal of Preventive and Social Medicine*', vol. 14, no. 1 (1960), pp. 9-15.

8. J.R. Ashford and M.G. Pearson, 'Who Uses the Health Services and Why?', *Journal of the Royal Statistical Society*, Series A (General), vol. 133, part 3 (1970), pp.295-345.

9. Office of Population Censuses and Surveys, Social Survey Division, *The General Household Survey, 1974* (HMSO, London, 1977), pp. 160, 164, 165.

10. Ibid., pp. 155, 157, 164, 165. Forster has calculated use/need ratios from the General Household Survey data for 1972. These ratios decrease with socioeconomic group when chronic sickness rates and average number of days of

restricted activity are used as criteria of need. D.P. Forster, 'Social Class Differences in Sickness and General Practitioner Consultations', *Health Trends*, vol. 8, no. 2 (May 1976), pp. 29-32.

11. Office of Population Censuses, *General Household Survey, 1975* (HMSO London, 1978), pp. 140, 142, 145.

12. Cartwright, *Patients and Their Doctors.*

13. Government Social Survey, *Diptheria Immunisation Inquiry*, by P.G. Gray and A. Cartwright (HMSO, London, 1952).

14. G.R. Osborn and V.N. Leyshon, 'Domiciliary Testing of Cervical Smears by Home Nurses', *Lancet*, i (1966), pp. 256-7.

15. Department of Health and Social Security, *The Multiple Health Screening Clinic, Rotherham, 1966: A Social and Economic Assessment*, by J.L. Girt, L.A. Hooper and R.A. Abel, Reports on Public Health and Medical Subjects, no. 121 (HMSO, London, 1969).

16. Ann Cartwright, *Parents and Family Planning Services* (Routledge and Kegan Paul, London, 1970).

17. Ibid., p. 46.

18. Ann Cartwright, *Human Relations and Hospital Care* (Routledge and Kegan Paul, London, 1964).

19. Ibid., p. 191.

20. Cartwright, *Patients and Their Doctors.*

21. Ibid., pp. 205-7.

22. S.J.L. Taylor, *Good General Practice* (Oxford University Press, London, 1954).

23. J.S. Collings, 'General Practice in England Today', *Lancet*, i (1950), pp. 555-85.

24. Taylor, *Good General Practice*, p. 38.

25. Ibid., p. 41.

26. Richard M. Titmuss, 'Role of the Family Doctor Today in the Context of Britain's Social Services', *Lancet*, i (1965), pp. 1-4.

27. Collings, 'General Practice in England Today'.

28. Cartwright, *Human Relations and Hospital Care*, p. 81; Ann Cartwright, 'What Goes on in the General Practitioner's Surgery?' in Roy M. Acheson and Lesley Aird (eds.), *Seminars in Community Medicine*, vol. 1, Sociology (Oxford University Press, London, 1976).

29. Taylor, *Good General Practice*, p. 40.

Access to NHS Hospital Care

If little attention has been paid to class patterns of use of general practitioner services, then patterns of hospitalisation have been almost ignored. Official data on hospital admissions and discharges do not generally indicate the social class of patients and there are relatively few studies which have been concerned with the class representation of hospital patients. To further cloud the issue, those studies which do provide us with information on class rates of hospitalisation point to different conclusions.

The most comprehensive and most recent study of hospital admissions is the Hospital Inpatient Enquiry for 1960 and 1961.[1] This is one of the few such inquiries which provides data on the social class of patients. Table 9.1 shows admissions, mean duration of stay, and percentage of beds used for each social class and for occupational groupings within classes III, IV, and V. Comparing the representation of the classes within the hospitals with the class distribution of males in England and Wales in 1961, we see that class IV and, particularly, class V, are proportionately over-represented. Class V has both high admission rates and longer than average periods of hospitalisation, and while classes IV and V represent 21 per cent and 9 per cent of the population, they occupy 26.5 per cent and 14.2 per cent respectively of hospital beds. This same pattern is evident in a study by Ashford and Pearson of thirty-five general practices in Exeter, which shows a marked tendency for the hospital admission rate to increase with decreasing social class; the difference between class I and class V was almost 50 per cent of the average of all classes.[2] A Political and Economic Planning survey also suggests that hospitals serve a larger proportion of working class than middle class patients.[3] Eighty-nine per cent of unskilled workers' families had at some time received treatment in an outpatient department and 84 per cent of the families of managerial and professional workers had done so. Hospital inpatient care had been given to 89 per cent of the former and 75 per cent of the latter.

But other studies suggest different conclusions. For example, Abel-Smith and Titmuss examined the class distribution among discharges from hospitals in England and Wales in 1949, and as Table 9.2 shows, the class distribution of men in each of the three types of hospital is very close to that in England and Wales, and, for the London teaching

Table 9.1: Admissions, Mean Duration of Stay and Percentage of Beds Used by Social Class, England and Wales, 1960-1

Social Class	Admissions in sample		Mean duration of stay (days)	Beds used %	England and Wales (males) 1961
	Under 65 %	All Ages %			
I Professional	2.3	2.4	17.3	1.9	4
II Intermediate	10.8	11.6	19.2	10.2	15
III Skilled workers	51.4	50.0		47.3	51
a) Mine workers (all types)	1.4	1.3	23.5	1.4	
b) Transport workers	5.8	5.5	19.9	5.0	
c) Clerical workers	7.4	7.4	20.1	6.7	
d) Armed forces	0.9	0.9	27.7	1.2	
e) Others	35.9	34.9	20.8	33.0	
IV Semi-skilled workers	22.9	23.2		26.5	21
a) Agricultural	2.2	2.4	39.3	4.4	
b) Others	20.7	20.8	23.3	22.1	
V Unskilled workers	12.6	12.8		14.2	9
a) Building & dock labourers	1.8	1.8	25.0	2.1	
b) Others	10.8	11.0	24.2	12.1	
Total	67,727	82,629	22.0	51,268	

Sources: Ministry of Health and General Register Office, *Report of Hospital Inpatient Enquiry for the Two Years 1960 and 1961*, Part III (HMSO, London, 1967), Table VI,8, p. 365. The social class distribution in England and Wales in 1961 is taken from D.C. Marsh, *The Changing Social Structure of England and Wales 1871-1961*, revised edn (Routledge and Kegan Paul, London, 1965) p. 198.

Table 9.2: Proportionate Distribution by Social Class of Discharges
in 1949 from Three Groups of Hospitals Participating in the General
Register Office's Study of Hospital Morbidity in England and Wales,
Males Aged 25-64 Years, All Diagnostic Conditions Excluding Injuries

Social Class	London Teaching Hospitals %	Provincial Teaching Hospitals %	Regional Board Hospitals %	England and Wales 1951 %	Greater London 1951 %
I and II	21	16	15	20	21
III	56	55	58	51	55
IV and V	23	29	27	29	24

Source: B. Abel-Smith and R.M. Titmuss, *The Cost of the National Health Service
in England and Wales* (Cambridge University Press, Cambridge, 1956), Table 88,
p. 149.

hospitals, to that in Greater London in 1951. But because of the higher
death rates and greater sickness of classes IV and V, we would expect
them to make greater demands on the hospital service and to be
proportionally over-represented within the hospital population. In consequence, Abel-Smith and Titmuss conclude that there is an inequality
of access to hospital care, in that working class patients are less likely to
be hospitalised than their needs for care would lead us to expect. The
differences between the national data for 1949 and those from the
Hospital Inpatient Enquiry for 1961 are not very great, but they do
suggest different conclusions and it may be the case that class patterns
of hospitalisation changed slightly over the period and in such a direction as to provide working class patients with easier access to care. For
example, the 1949 data may reflect the fact that middle class patients
had just been provided with easy access to hospitals as a result of the
introduction of the NHS. For a period of time, therefore, they may
have been receiving treatment which they had been unable to obtain
in earlier years, but once this 'backlog' was cleared, they made fewer
demands on the hospital service. However, there are several smaller scale
studies which suggest that there continues to be inequality in the use of
hospital services in certain areas, if not on a national scale.

Barr's study of hospital admissions in April and May 1956 sought to
determine whether admission rates were linked with the quality of
social environment.[4] The data refer to the area served by the group of
four hospitals in the county borough of Reading and four indices were
used to assess the social environment — the social class distribution,
persons per household, density per room, and the proportion of persons

with the exclusive use of piped water, a water closet, stove, sink, and bath. Standardised hospital admission ratios for each sex and speciality were correlated with each of these social indices and there was some evidence that admission rates increased as environment improved, with most of the significant correlations occurring in traumatic and ortho-paedic surgery and gynaecology specialities. Barr points out that the degree of correlation in many instances was not great, but that, never-theless, the results were reasonably consistent.

Similar findings have also been obtained by Airth and Newell in the Hartlepools and Tees-side in 1957-8.[5] The authors expected to find higher admission rates in areas with poor living conditions, because poor health forces people into, or keeps them in such areas, and because these living conditions can give rise to ill-health. They took the number of persons per room in the study areas as an index of living conditions and this had a strong negative association with the proportion of persons in classes I and II in the areas. Class A areas (with fewer than 0.61 persons per room) produced nearly 2 per cent more hospital cases per 1,000 population than Class E areas (with over 0.92 persons per room), and the difference between the areas became more marked when specialities with widely variable durations of stay were excluded. But the pattern changed when length of hospitalisation was taken into account. For all specialities, Class E areas required 30 per cent more bed-days per head than Class A areas and, excluding long stay special-ities, the excess was 10 per cent. A case admitted from a Class E district stayed, on average, one-third as long again as one from Class A districts. For restricted specialities, the difference was 15 per cent. This suggests that middle class patients are slightly more likely to be admitted to hospital, but that they have a shorter period of hospitalisation.

Two studies by Alderson also indicate an under-representation of working class patients in the hospital population. One, a study of patients who died from cancer in April 1969 and who were resident in the county borough of Manchester, shows that semi and unskilled manual workers were more likely to be nursed at home.[6] However, the numbers are small and the differences not significant. The other is a study of a representative sample of adults who died in Bristol between October 1962 and September 1963.[7] Of the 2,243 deaths, 26 per cent had not been referred to hospital for either investigation or treatment, and if deaths from neoplasms (where the vast majority attended hospital), sudden deaths, and those from coronary disease (where death is unexpected) are excluded, 29 per cent of the total had not been referred to hospital. The percentages rose from 24 per cent in classes I and II to 36 per cent in class V.

We may also note a reluctance on the part of some working class women to have their babies delivered in hospital. A study by Butler and Bonham of perinatal mortality among mothers giving birth between 3 and 9 March 1958 in England and Wales, indicates that married women in classes IV and V are most likely to plan to have their children at home, even though more complications are likely to arise at birth.[8] Women in classes I and II, and unmarried women are most likely to arrange to have their children in hospital or a general practitioner unit. But these differences are not so pronounced for actual deliveries since a higher proportion of women have their children in hospital than plan to do so. Consequently, though there are still marked class variations in the proportion of births taking place at home or in a general practitioner unit, there are only small differences in the proportions of hospital births; mothers in class I are just slightly more likely than mothers from other social classes to give birth in hospital. Mothers in class I are also more likely than mothers in other social classes to receive all their prenatal care from a hospital.

Finally, there is some evidence of other types of class differences in Titmuss's study of blood donors.[9] In addition to tabulating the social class of blood donors, he presents figures on the social class of recipients of blood transfusions. The number of recipients of blood increases with social class, with the differences being most marked among men; the percentage excess of classes I and II over classes IV and V is 120 per cent for men and 35 per cent for women. He concludes that these data signify real class differences — that higher social classes receive more blood transfusions and surgical operations or other medical treatments calling for blood. He comments:

> This is an unexpected finding. The whole weight of evidence on the social class incidence of mortality and morbidity, of industrial accidents and to a large extent road accidents, and of the risks of childbearing among mothers with large families from poor homes would have indicated contrary results. In short, we would have expected — particularly under a free National Health Service — to find that, taking account of these factors, blood transfusions would be relatively more numerous among S.C. IV-V.[10]

No explanation of the differences is offered by the author, but it is important to note that these data are based on a survey of blood donors — we know nothing of the experience of people who have not given blood. It is, therefore, unwise to generalise from these observations, even though there appears to be no marked class bias in the persons donating blood.

Thus, most of the information which is available to us suggests inequality in the use of hospital services. But we cannot readily conclude that working class patients are disadvantaged in access to care. In the first place, we need more national data on the social class of patients admitted to hospital and their lengths of stay. We also need more studies which chart the careers of patients of different social classes — studies which explore class differences in the recognition of symptoms, ways of coping with these, the stages at which professional advice is sought and the action which follows from this. Only with the understanding that such studies might provide, can we interpret the significance of national statistics. For high rates of hospitalisation among working class patients can be interpreted in different ways. On the one hand, they may be taken to indicate that patients have easy access to general practitioners and that, whenever necessary, they are referred for hospital treatment. On the other hand, such high rates have been seen to reflect a situation in which, as a result of lack of access to primary care, consultations take place at a later and more serious stage in illness, when there is a greater need for hospitalisation.[11] In other words, high admission rates for working class patients can be taken to represent either equality of access to care or quite the opposite. In order to assess the nature and extent of class inequalities in access to care, we need some understanding of class difference in the careers of patients, for we cannot interpret data on hospitalisation without reference to primary care. In the absence of such information, it is difficult to appreciate the significance of the data which are presently available to us.

Quality of Care

One important index of quality is whether or not patients are admitted to teaching hospitals: care in a non-teaching hospital may often be inferior to that in a teaching hospital, for the latter have 37 per cent more consultants, six times as many senior registrars, 56 per cent more registrars, 171 per cent more house officers, and 60 per cent more full-time nurses.[12] Moreover, differences in case-fatality ratios between teaching and non-teaching hospitals imply that the two types of hospitals may be providing different standards of care:

There is no doubt that patients of comparable age, sex, and social class stand a much higher chance of dying in a non-teaching hospital from conditions such as appendicitis with peritonitis, hyperplasia of the prostrate, ischaemic heart disease, skull fracture and other head injuries, and a number of other common causes of hospital admission . . . the gap between the two types of hospital is by no means narrowing over the years.[13]

It is not clear whether there are differences in the proportions of different social classes within the two types of hospital; Cartwright found no class differences in whether patients were admitted to a teaching or non-teaching hospital,[14] yet Ashley *et al.* found that within the same catchment area, a teaching hospital may attract or select the more advantaged.[15] This latter study of local admissions from a district in which both types of hospitals were situated shows that 46 per cent of the patients in the regional board hospital belonged to classes IV and V, while only 33 per cent of those in the teaching hospital did so. A similar difference was not found in the other three hospitals included in the study. Clearly, as with several other issues we have touched on, further research is needed in this area. As the authors indicate:

Why this should be so after twenty years of the National Health Service is one of the seemingly innumerable questions that can be asked about the loose — even random — matching of needs and resources in the medical and social services. For a start, nobody seemed to have the facts.[16]

As far as other indices of quality are concerned, there appear to be no class differences. Cartwright's study of hospital patients indicates that there were no class differences in delays in admission to hospital; in the proportions visited at home by a consultant; in facilities such as curtains, screens, telephones, visiting times, and the hours at which patients were woken in the morning; in the proportions of surgical patients who had seen the surgeon and anaesthetist; and in the size of the ward.[17] In fact, only one major difference between classes emerged in her study of hospital care and she summarises this as follows:

The most striking class difference is in the amount of financial hardship experienced by patients who normally worked. In this respect we are indeed two nations, one receiving full wages or salary from their employers, the other reduced to the penury of national insurance sickness benefit.[18]

While it is difficult to reach any firm conclusions about the access of working class patients to NHS hospital care, there is, nevertheless, an institutionalised class inequality within the hospital system, for the National Health Service Act of 1946 guaranteed the continued existence of private health care.[19] Though private beds in NHS hospitals are now being phased out, the number of beds in private hospitals is steadily increasing. Only a small proportion of the population has availed itself of these services, but the demand for private care, particularly private hospital care, is increasing.

Private Hospital Care

Private Medical Care Schemes

With the introduction of the NHS, contributory and provident societies were faced with a threat to their continued existence. While contributory schemes were associated with the working class, provident societies catered to the middle class. The former turned to providing mainly sickness benefits to their members (such as cash benefits during a period of hospitalisation, and contributions toward glasses, dentures, and surgical appliances) while the provident associations focused their efforts on insuring their members against the costs of private hospital care.[20] Thus their class role was duplicated after 1948. Only a small proportion of the population has opted to pay for private health care, yet the private system is important, not for its extensiveness, but for its symbolic significance and for the threat which it poses for the quality of care available under the NHS. The continued provision of private care is an affirmation of class inequality, for it guarantees the existence of two levels of care and gives the right to patients who have the money, to pay for privileges.

The British United Provident Association (BUPA) was formed in 1947 and soon amalgamated with several existing provident associations. It now has a virtual monopoly of the market and in 1977, it received 74 per cent of the total subscription income from all provident schemes. Private Patients Plan is the second largest with 23 per cent of total subscription income.[21] Membership in these schemes has grown considerably and after an annual increase during the 1960s of between 7.5 and 8 per cent, the total number of subscribers reached 883,000 in 1969.[22] By 1976, there were over 1,057,000 subscribers.[23] There is little detailed information on the types of patients who choose private medical care, though one survey shows that in 1966, BUPA's membership was disproportionately composed of older, highly paid married men approaching the end of their careers who were members of group or company schemes. Only two per cent of the membership were manual workers while 37 per cent were employed in professional and managerial occupations.[24]

Group schemes account for a high proportion of the membership increase. Between 1964 and 1976, individual subscriptions increased by 4 per cent while group subscriptions rose by 113 per cent. In 1976, 74 per cent of subscriptions were on a group basis compared to only 58 per cent in 1964. BUPA policy has been directed towards attracting members on a group basis; it has allowed a 20 per cent reduction for groups where a company sponsors the scheme, but does not contribute to the cost; a 25 per cent reduction where the company contributes half or more of the cost; and a 33.33 per cent reduction where the whole cost of membership in a scheme is borne by the company. The companies can, in turn, claim their payments into such schemes as a tax deductible business expense, which can reduce their costs by a further 40 per cent.[25] Mencher notes that:

> the advantage of this appeal over that to individuals is that it avoids the controversial issue of individual preference and preferred treat-ment in a democratic welfare society. By placing the onus on the firm's need, private insurance becomes the handmaiden of efficiency and higher productivity and enhances social rather than individual goals.[26]

The growth of these provident schemes is a measure of the vitality of private practice and it can act as a stimulus to further growth. Their growth convinces people of the inherent advantages of private care, and conversely, of the limitations of care within the NHS. At present the private health sector cannot exist without access to the facilities of the NHS; approximately 60-70 per cent of BUPA patients are treated in NHS hospitals, the remainder in private hospitals and nursing homes.[27] But in these private hospitals there may be the seeds of an independent, parallel hospital service. BUPA has a virtual monopoly of the privately controlled hospitals and other facilities outside the NHS and it is building small hospitals with about thirty beds and full X-ray, theatre and diagnostic facilities at the rate of two or three a year. There is now a total of 900 beds in such private hospitals and the number should reach 1,000 in 1979. But the future may bring significant changes in the

rate of growth of such facilities and the nature of their funding —
especially with the phasing out of private beds in NHS hospitals and a
deterioration in the care available to NHS patients. A BUPA spokesman
comments:

> Increasingly as the demand for these places grows, I am looking in
> economic terms at whether it would be advisable to go to the
> market and raise capital and pay interest on it, and try running in
> parallel, particularly in the London area, with hospitals which were
> entirely there on a non-profit, but certainly commercial basis, where
> we would have full control.[28]

The Effect of Private Health Care on the NHS

Why do people seek private hospital care? The main reasons appear to
be the opportunities to choose the time of hospitalisation; to receive
care more quickly than NHS patients (in non-urgent cases); to choose
one's consultant and be sure that he will perform any operations; to
have more attention paid to medical tests (which have the consultant's
name on them); and a feeling that one will generally receive better
service and attention.[29] Arguments have been advanced that NHS
patients are deprived of the care which they should be receiving as a
result of the demands made by private patients on hospital facilities and
on consultants, and these arguments gained such prominence that in
1970-1, the House of Commons' Employment and Social Services Sub-
committee conducted hearings on the use of NHS facilities by private
patients. The minutes of evidence of this committee provide numerous
examples of the ways in which the treatment of NHS patients suffers
because priority is frequently given to private patients. The report of
the Expenditure Committee summarises a part of this evidence as
follows:

> Though the number of beds approved for private use are required to
> be made available to National Health Service patients if not in use,
> it was alleged that it was 'not uncommon for beds to be wasted
> because they are being kept empty for private admissions'. Also, it
> was added that because of long waiting lists for some types of
> surgical treatment, private patients obtained preferential admissions
> to National Health Service hospitals for surgical treatment, which
> meant National Health Service patients had to wait longer. It was
> stated that National Health Service patients who should be nursed in
> single rooms, for medical reasons, may be kept in large wards or

moved into large wards so that private patients may obtain the privacy paid for. Other statements concerned the preferential use of operating theatres and diagnostic facilities. It was said that when private patients were included in the National Health Service operating sessions, they were usually placed early in the list so that operations on National Health Service patients 'with an equal or superior priority' might be delayed or even cancelled. Regarding diagnoses such as special radiological investigations, it was asserted that though patients would be booked for specific times long in advance, if a private patient were brought in at short notice, it 'usually led to the cancellation of one or more National Health Service appointments'.[30]

Evidence was also presented of NHS beds being used by private patients;[31] of a lowering of staff morale due to consultants' neglect of their NHS work and excessive delegation of responsibility of such patients to juniors;[32] and of specific abuses such as the theft or borrowing of medical equipment and expensive instruments for private work.[33] But the many such examples of threats to the quality of NHS care due to the demands of private practice were given only token recognition by the Expenditure Committee. Albeit by a narrow majority, their conclusions were

that private practice operates to the overall benefit of the National Health Service. We recognise that, from time to time, abuses may occur as they may in any large organisation. We do not condone this situation, but we do not believe abuses to be widespread or of any magnitude.[34]

Such a conclusion is hardly surprising if we consider, not only the interests of patients who can afford to pay for private care, but also those of consultants. Certainly the evidence of consultants appearing before the Expenditure Committee was supportive of existing arrangements for private practice. The combination of private and NHS work can be lucrative; in 1955-6, the average income of part-time male consultants in Britain was £3,603 while that of full-time consultants was £3,002, and the average income of those in the highest income decile of part-time workers was £5,393 while their full-time counterparts received an average of £3,782.[35] The 1974 Review Body on Doctors' and Dentists' Remuneration estimated that, compounded between the ages of 37 and 64 years, work outside the NHS was worth £75,735 to consultants working on a part-time basis.[36] Any restrictions on consultants' rights to enter private practice would, therefore, lower their income considerably and might cause many to leave the country. The Report of the Expenditure Committee did recognise the role played by private practice in keeping top consultants in Britain, but it failed to recognise the implications of a continued growth of private practice for the NHS.

The continued growth of the private sector can have an increasing impact on the quality of care received within the public sector. In order for a demand for private care to exist, it has to provide benefits not available under the NHS, and its existence can contribute to the further deterioration of public care. This circular process could easily accelerate when NHS hospitals face cutbacks, shortages of staff and strikes — each of which may lead to delays in treatment. By attracting mainly middle class patients, private schemes rob the NHS of its most vocal and critical patients — patients whose continued use of NHS hospitals might otherwise help to generate improvements within the public service. Thus the continued growth of provident schemes serves to convince people that they do have something to offer, and as they continue to prosper, the public service deteriorates.

The existence of a private health sector bestows the opportunity on patients who can afford to do so, to pay for privileges which are by no means simply non-medical privileges. Thus, recognition is given to the distribution of medical care on a basis other than need and to the availability of two levels of care. As Mencher comments, 'Since the rationale for private practice, when free medical care is available to all, must largely imply some service, the question of private practice cannot be comfortably divorced from the provision of two standards of care'.[37] In fact, the NHS appears to have achieved little change; just as before 1948, the wealthy can pay for private care while workers receive public care. It is true that the majority of people receive public care, but a privilege has been retained — one which appears to be increasingly attractive to middle class patients. Continued growth of the private sector could produce two parallel health services; one catering largely to the middle class, the other to the working class.

Conclusion

While it is not altogether clear whether working class patients are disadvantaged in their access to NHS hospitals, the availability of private health care represents the institutionalisation of class inequalities in access to hospital care. The opportunity for patients to pay for private care has been interpreted as an opportunity for them to obtain non-medical benefits which are not available under the NHS. Viewed in this light, the existence of the private sector does not challenge the belief that medical care is provided on the basis of need alone. Yet there is evidence to suggest that private care also bestows medical privileges and that the growth of the private sector may threaten the quality of care available within the NHS. Indeed, if the private sector continues to expand, it may be meaningless to ask whether working class patients have equal access to care under the NHS, for these hospitals could become essentially working class institutions. The introduction of the NHS has served the interests of middle class patients; not only have they been able to take full advantage of NHS hospital care, they have retained the right to pay for private care and the medical privileges which it brings. Moreover, private hospital patients are no longer confined to smaller hospitals providing inferior care. In effect, middle class patients benefited from the introduction of socialised medicine, and saw an extension of the benefits attached to receiving private care.

Notes

1. Ministry of Health and General Register Office, *Reports of Hospital Inpatient Enquiry for the Two Years 1960 and 1961*, part III (HMSO, London, 1967).

2. J.R. Ashford and M.G. Pearson, 'Who Uses the Health Services and Why?' *Journal of the Royal Statistical Society*, Series A (General), vol. 133, part 3 (1970), pp. 295-345.

3. Political and Economic Planning, *Family Needs and the Social Services* (Allen and Unwin, London, 1961), pp. 55-7.

4. A. Barr, 'Hospital Admissions and Social Environment', *The Medical Officer*, vol. 100, no. 23 (1958), pp. 351-4.

5. A.D. Airth and D.J. Newell, *The Demand for Hospital Beds* (University of Durham, King's College, Newcastle-upon-Tyne, 1962).

6. M.R. Alderson, 'Terminal Care in Malignant Disease', *British Journal of Preventive and Social Medicine*, vol. 24, no. 2 (1970), pp. 120-3.

7. M.R. Alderson, 'Referral to Hospital Among a Representative Sample of Adults Who Died', *Proceedings of the Royal Society of Medicine*, vol. 59, no. 2 (1966), pp. 719-21.

8. N.R. Butler and D.G. Bonham, *Perinatal Mortality* (E. and S. Livingstone, London, 1963).

9. R.M. Titmuss, *The Gift Relationship* (Allen and Unwin, London, 1970).

10. Ibid., p. 136.

11. R. Andersen *et al.*, *Medical Care Use in Sweden and the U.S.* (University of Chicago Press, Chicago, 1970).

12. G. Forsyth, *Doctors and State Medicine: A Study of the British Health Service* (Pitman Medical Publishing Co. Ltd, London, 1966).

13. Ibid., p. 97.

14. Ann Cartwright, *Human Relations and Hospital Care* (Routledge and

Kegan Paul, London, 1964).

15. J.S.A. Ashley *et al.*, 'Case Fatality of Hyperplasia of the Prostrate in Two Teaching and Three Regional Board Hospitals', *Lancet*, ii (1971), pp. 1308-11.

16. Ibid., p. 1311.

17. Cartwright, *Human Relations and Hospital Care.*

18. Ibid., p. 202.

19. Of course, it is not only in the hospital system that the private care is available, but the demand is greater for hospital care, where delays are most likely to be experienced by patients. About 2-3 per cent of patients receive private care from general practitioners, but we have no data on the social class of these patients, the use they make of GPs and the quality of care they receive. D.S. Lees, 'Private General Practice and the National Health Service', *Sociological Review*, Monograph no. 5 (July 1962), pp. 33-47.

20. B. Abel-Smith, *The Hospitals 1800-1948* (Heinemann, London, 1964), pp. 401-2.

21. *U.K. Private Medical Care:Provident Schemes Statistics, 1977* (Lee Donaldson Associates, London, 1978).

22. M. Lee, *Opting Out of the National Health Service* (Political and Economic Planning, London, 1971), p. 13.

23. *U.K. Private Medical Care: Provident Schemes Statistics, 1976* (Lee Donaldson Associates, London, 1977), p. 10.

24. Lee, *Opting Out of the NHS*, p. 16.

25. House of Commons, Expenditure Committee, *National Health Service Facilities for Private Patients* (HMSO, London, 1972), p. 35.

26. S. Mencher, *Private Practice in Britain* (G. Bell and Sons, London, 1967), p. 30.

27. House of Commons, *NHS Facilities for Private Patients*, p. 36.

28. Ibid., p. 47.

29. Mencher, *Private Practice in Britain*, Ch. 3.

30. House of Commons, *NHS Facilities for Private Patients*, p. xvi.

31. Ibid., p. xxi.

32. Ibid., p. xvii.

33. Ibid., p. xviii.

34. Ibid., p. xxii.

35. Mencher, *Private Practice in Britain*, p. 19.

36. Review Body on Doctors' and Dentists' Remuneration, *Fourth Report, 1974*, Comd. 5644 (HMSO, London, 1974), p. 42.

37. Mencher, *Private Practice in Britain*, p. 73.

10 CONCLUSION

The NHS has commonly been understood as a response to the poorer health and access to care of working class patients. It is often argued that the growth of social welfare legislation in general, and the introduction of the NHS in particular, stems from the conflict arising from class inequalities. As such, social reforms are viewed as an attempt on the part of the state to diffuse class conflict by improving the situation of the working class. Yet the success of the NHS in providing equal access to health care has seldom been questioned. Initially, the service was regarded with something close to veneration and while it has received more critical attention in recent years, few studies have explored the nature and extent of class inequalities within the health sector. Given the universal provision of health care at no direct cost, it is assumed that the service distributes care on the basis of need alone and that social class differences in the consumption of health services have virtually disappeared.[1]

The data I have reviewed suggest that these interpretations of the introduction and impact of the NHS are inappropriate. As far as the introduction of the service is concerned, there is little evidence that working class patients were singularly disadvantaged in their access to medical care before 1948 and working class pressures for reform were neither strong nor did they envisage comprehensive changes in the organisation and delivery of health care. The two main representatives of the organised working class — the Trades Union Congress and the Labour Party — were concerned with reform of the health services during the inter-war years, but these concerns were given only sporadic expression and it was not until the early forties that the two organisations were committed to the idea of a comprehensive reorganisation of the health sector. They were responding to, rather than initiating the debate over reform. Even if we take a broader index of class conflict — strike activity — then there is little evidence of the radicalisation of the working class.[2] In consequence, it is difficult to interpret the introduction of the NHS as a response to working class demands for reform.

Instead, I have argued that the state was responding to the organisational and fiscal problems within the health sector and that it was seeking to create a rational, efficient, nationally co-ordinated health service. These problems became increasingly severe during the twenties

156

and thirties and they were both highlighted and exacerbated by the demands placed on the services during wartime. The organisation and delivery of health care was deficient in several respects; duplication of services; maldistribution of resources; shortages of personnel and facilities; minimal co-ordination between the numerous units providing and financing care; fiscal crises within the voluntary hospital system; deficiencies in the National Health Insurance scheme; and problems which middle class patients faced in financing treatment and obtaining access to adequate hospital care. All these problems signified a poorly organised, inadequately financed and inefficient health care system.

The proposals for change which were advanced by different branches of the medical profession, as well as the explanations of the need for reform which were provided by both the Conservative and Labour parties, show a concern with resolving these organisational problems. The proposals of the different professional bodies varied in details, as did the changes planned by both parties, but there was a consistency in the problems which were identified and in the recognition of a need for a nationally co-ordinated state medical service. In all instances, the major goal was the creation of a rational, efficient health service and this was to be achieved through an extension of the state's responsibility in organising and financing medical care. The introduction of a national health service promised to improve care by redistributing resources, making more efficient use of these and providing a guaranteed source of funding for the health sector. At the same time, it promised to improve the incomes and working conditions of general practitioners and consultants, without necessarily threatening their professional autonomy.

It is difficult to determine the impact of the NHS. As a result of the widespread belief that the service distributed care on the basis of need alone, few studies have assessed its effectiveness in meeting the needs for care of working class and middle class patients. Yet there is evidence which challenges the general complacency as to the success with which the service provides equal access to care. The available data do not confirm the belief that the NHS increased the ease and frequency with which working class patients obtained medical care. Though the evidence is confusing and at times points to different conclusions, several studies also suggest that working class patients make less use of health services than their needs for care lead us to expect. Moreover, there is some evidence that the care they receive is of lesser quality than that obtained by middle class patients. In fact, middle class patients experienced several benefits as a result of the introduction of the service; for the first time they obtained care at no direct cost and they gained access to the major hospitals, while retaining the opportunity to pay for private care. Though the data leave much to be desired, it would be difficult to conclude that working class patients were the main beneficiaries of the NHS. We may also note that, despite the introduction of the National Health Insurance scheme and then the NHS, class inequalities in mortality rates have not diminished since the turn of the century.

If the NHS was not a response to class conflict and if it has achieved little reduction in class inequalities in health and access to care, then how can we conceptualise the role of the state? One response is consistent with a pluralistic image of contemporary industrial society. This perspective argues that the state serves the 'national interest' by mediating between classes and interest groups and ensuring that no one class or interest group dominates at the expense of others.[3] Even though the growth of social welfare legislation has often been seen as a response to class conflict, my thesis that the NHS was an attempt to rationalise the organisation and delivery of medical care can be incorporated within this pluralist model. It is consistent with this model to argue that the NHS was the state's response to problems which the medical profession in particular, identified within the health sector. The introduction of the service could thus be seen as one instance of the state functioning in a co-ordinating capacity and seeking to improve the provision of medical care.

It is this type of image of contemporary industrial society which is implicit in most of the research and writing on the organisation and delivery of health care. The emphasis is on a 'social engineering' approach, in which the state apparatus assumes responsibility for planning and co-ordinating the different units within the health sector. Problems such as class inequalities in health and access to care tend to be defined as problems of planning. It is assumed that deficiencies in the health care system can be resolved by further rationalising the organisation and delivery of health care; the problem is one of planning and obtaining the necessary information on which to base plans.[4] As far as patients are concerned, the problem is defined as one of changing the knowledge, values and life styles of working class patients. These are seen as capable of rational solution through the education of patients. The issues of illness and use of health services are thus reduced to individual dimensions, linked with the values and behaviour of individual patients.

The problem with this type of interpretation is that it tends to

Cultural / Behavioural
* due to cultural deprivation ?

isolate the health care sector and the issue of health from their broader social and political context. It is true that the social bases of illness are more frequently being recognised; with the growing prevalence of chronic diseases, the dangers of the life styles and social environment characteristic of industrial society are being acknowledged and our attention is drawn to the deleterious effects of poor nutrition, smoking, lack of exercise, stress and pollution. Thus the social costs of industrial-isation are starting to be recognised. But the responsibility for counter-acting the effects of industrialisation is still placed frequently on the shoulders of individuals. We are urged to change our life styes — to stop smoking and exercise more frequently, for example — and it is argued that considerable improvements in the health of individuals are likely to result from such changes in individual behaviour.[5] Yet little recog-nition is given to the limits of the changes which we can achieve while maintaining the structure of relations in an industrial capitalist society.

Also, there is little acknowledgement of the fact that the social costs of industrialisation are unequally distributed. We may recall that since the turn of the century at least, class inequalities in mortality rates have not diminished. Though life expectancy has increased throughout all classes, it has increased less rapidly in the working class. Moreover, morbidity rates indicate that illness and disability are more pervasive features of the life of the working class. What these consistent class inequalities suggest is that we should be looking beyond the general life styles characteristic of industrial society and exploring the links between illness and the nature of class relations in British society. Contrary to the beliefs of many, in the emergence of a middle class society class inequalities have not withered away and the social costs of capitalism are still borne unequally.[6] Poverty, exposure to occupational health hazards, alienating work, pollution and poor housing conditions have all been linked with illness and can help to explain the greater morbidity and higher mortality rates within the working class.[7] Yet health has seldom been defined as a political issue; the individual is held responsible for his or her health, despite the fact that individuals alone can do little to remove many of those factors which help to create illness.

Rather than addressing the social and political bases of health, the state has defined health largely as a problem of the distribution of health care. In planning the NHS, the state implicitly defined health in terms of access to curative care, while also giving some recognition to the importance of preventive medicine. In so doing, it adopted medical models of disease which emphasise physiologically based disease and in which illness is seen to be cured through medical intervention. As several writers have indicated, this is only one of several possible models which explain illness and define appropriate treatments.[8] Medicine is socially created and not grounded in some absolute scientific truth. Modern medicine is consistent with the broader capitalist environment, for it directs our attention away from the political bases of illness. It generally fails to address the health denying effects of such things as poverty, pollution, competitiveness, alienating work and job insecurity and it does not explore the links between these and the structure of class relations in British society. By adopting current medical defini- tions and presenting health as an issue of access to care, rather than as a political problem, the state has posed no challenge to the existing class structure and has had the effect of legitimising existing class in- equalities. Moreover, because the NHS removed the direct costs of care and, in theory, provided care to all people irrespective of their means, it gave rise to the notion that class inequalities in health would diminish. In these ways the state has served an ideological function, in that it has helped to create a belief in the decline of class inequalities and per- mitted an interpretation of continuing inequalities in terms which emphasise the individual's responsibility for his or her own health.

It is not clear whether the state can move beyond this legitimating role and provide solutions to people's health problems. At present, more medical intervention does not appear to be the answer. A more effective attack on illness may require that the state intervene in the process of capital accumulation, for it would require a reorganisation of the economy and the life styles associated with it. This would necessitate the removal of such things as occupational health hazards, industrial pollutants, nutritionally inadequate food products, unsafe commod- ities, alienating work and disparities in income, job security and standards of living. What this means is that 'human' concerns would be given priority over efficiency and the maximisation of output and profit. Until now, the state has shown relatively little commitment to such priorities. Whether and under which conditions, it can assume such a role remains to be seen.

To summarise, I have argued that the NHS represented an attempt on the part of the state to rationalise the organisation and delivery of health care. In so doing, the state defined health largely in terms of access to care and by claiming to provide universal access to care, it has contributed to the belief that class inequalities in health and access to care have virtually disappeared. The strength of this belief is witnessed by the general complacency as to the success of the service in providing care on the basis of need alone and by the relative absence of research which explores the links between health, the organisation and delivery of health care and the nature of class relations in British society. This suggests that the state has served an ideological function insofar as it has legitimised medical definitions of health and failed to address class inequalities in health and the political bases of these. Hopefully, the future will see more research which focuses on these issues.

Notes

1. Charges have been introduced for some goods and services but low income patients can claim exemption from these charges. Also, the availability of private medical care has generally been interpreted as an opportunity for patients to pay for non-medical privileges. Thus, it has been assumed that patients' payments will neither reduce their use of services nor guarantee superior treatment.

2. It is possible that the anticipation of post-war class conflict led the state to introduce social reforms, but it is difficult to test this thesis.

3. It is argued that the class domination which characterises capitalism has been transcended in advanced industrial societies. Insofar as classes are recognised in such 'post-capitalist' societies, they are identified on the basis of supposedly marginal differences in income, consumption and prestige. See, for example, J. Strachey, *Contemporary Capitalism* (Victor Gollancz, London, 1956); D. Jay, *Socialism in the New Society* (Longmans, London, 1962).

4. For an example of this emphasis on systematic planning see Robert Kohn and Kerr L. White, *Health Care: An International Study* (Oxford University Press, London, 1976).

5. Such arguments can be founded in Ivan Illich, *Limits to Medicine* (McClelland and Stewart, Toronto, 1976); Marc Lalonde, *A New Perspective on the Health of Canadians* (Information Canada, Ottawa, 1975); Saxon Graham, 'Social Factors in Relation to the Chronic Illnesses' in H.E. Freeman, S. Levine and L.G. Reeder (eds.), *Handbook of Medical Sociology* (Prentice-Hall, Englewood Cliffs, New Jersey, 1972). This perspective has been criticised in Vicente Navarro, 'The Industrialization of Fetishism or the Fetishism of Industrialization: A Critique of Ivan Illich', *Social Science and Medicine*, vol. 9 (1975), pp. 351-63 and Marc Renaud, 'On the Structural Constraints to State Intervention in Health', *International Journal of Health Services*, vol. 5, no. 4 (1975), pp. 559-71.

6. For a critique of the notion that class domination no longer exists and that class inequalities have virtually disappeared in British society, see John Westergaard and Henrietta Resler, *Class in a Capitalist Society* (Penguin, Harmondsworth, 1976).

7. Joseph Eyer and Peter Sterling, 'Stress Related Mortality and Social Organization' *The Review of Radical Political Economics*, vol. 9, no. 1 (1977), pp. 1-44; James S. House, 'The Effects of Occupational Stress on Physical Health' in James O'Toole (ed.), *Work and the Quality of Life* (MIT Press, Cambridge, Mass., 1974); Elliott A. Krause, *Power and Illness: The Political Sociology of Health and Medical Care* (Elsevier, New York, 1977), Ch. 9; T. McKeown and C.R. Lowe, *An Introduction to Social Medicine*, 2nd edn (Blackwell, Oxford, 1974), Chs. 11, 16, 17, 18.

8. Hans Peter Dreitzel (ed.), *The Social Organisation of Health* (Macmillan, New

York, 1971), pp. v-xvii; Eliot Friedson, *Profession of Medicine: A Study of the Sociology of Applied Knowledge* (Harper and Row, New York, 1970); M. Rossdale, 'Health in a Sick Society', *New Left Review*, no. 34 (1965), pp. 82-91.

BIBLIOGRAPHY

'A Plan for British Hospitals', *Lancet*, ii (1939), pp. 945-51

Abel-Smith, Brian. *The Hospitals 1800-1948* (Heinemann, London, 1964)

—— and Richard M. Titmuss. *The Cost of the National Health Service in England and Wales* (Cambridge University Press, Cambridge, 1956)

Airth, A.D. and Newell, D.J. *The Demand for Hospital Beds* (University of Durham, King's College, Newcastle-upon-Tyne, 1962)

Alderson, M.R. 'Terminal Care in Malignant Disease.' *British Journal of Preventive and Social Medicine*, vol. 24, no. 2 (1970), pp. 120-3

——. 'Referral to Hospital Among a Representative Sample of Adults Who Died', *Proceedings of the Royal Society of Medicine*, vol. 59, no. 2 (1966), pp. 719-21

Andersen, R., *et al*. *Medical Care Use in Sweden and the U.S.* (University of Chicago Press, Chicago, 1970)

Ashford, J.R. and Pearson, M.G. 'Who Uses the Health Services and Why?', *Journal of the Royal Statistical Society*, Series A (General), vol. 133, part 3 (1970), pp. 295-345

Ashley, J.S.A. *et al*. 'Case Fatality of Hyperplasia of the Prostate in Two Teaching and Three Regional Board Hospitals', *Lancet*, ii (1971), pp. 1308-11

Badgley, Robin F. and Wolfe, Samuel. *Doctors Strike: Medical Care and Conflict in Saskatchewan* (Macmillan of Canada, Toronto, 1967).

Barr, A. 'Hospital Admissions and Social Environment', *The Medical Officer*, vol. 100, no. 23 (1958), pp. 351-4

Bendix, R. *Work and Authority in Industry* (Harper and Row, New York, 1963)

Beveridge, Sir William. *Report on Social Insurance and Allied Services* (HMSO, London, 1942)

Birnbaum, N. *The Crisis of Industrial Society* (Oxford University Press, London, 1969)

Brand, Jeanne L. *Doctors and the State: The British Medical Profession and Government Action in Public Health, 1870-1912* (The Johns Hopkins Press, Baltimore, 1965)

British Hospitals Association. *Report of the Voluntary Hospitals Commission* (British Hospitals Association, London, 1937)

British Institute of Public Opinion. *The Beveridge Report and the Public*

(British Institute of Public Opinion, London, n.d.)

British Medical Association. *A General Medical Service for the Nation* (British Medical Association, London, 1938)

——. *Proposals for a General Medical Service for the Nation* (British Medical Association, London, 1929)

Bruce, M. *The Coming of the Welfare State* (B.T. Batsford, London, 1966)

Butler, N.R. and Bonham, D.G. *Perinatal Mortality* (E. and S. Livingstone, London, 1963)

Cartwright, Ann. 'What Goes on in the General Practitioner's Surgery?' in Roy M. Acheson and Lesley Aird (eds.), *Seminars in Community Medicine*, vol. I, Sociology (Oxford University Press, London, 1976)

——. *Parents and Family Planning Services* (Routledge and Kegan Paul, London, 1970)

——. *Patients and Their Doctors: A Study of General Practice* (Routledge and Kegan Paul, London, 1967)

——. *Human Relations and Hospital Care* (Routledge and Kegan Paul, London, 1964)

—— and O'Brien, Maureen.'Social Class Variations in Health Care and in the Nature of General Practitioner Consultations' in M. Stacey (ed.), *The Sociology of the NHS*, Sociological Review Monograph, no. 22 (University of Keele, Keele, 1976)

Central Statistical Office. 'The Incidence of Taxes and Social Service Benefits in 1963 and 1964', *Economic Trends*, no. 154 (August 1966), pp. i-ix

Cochrane, A.L. *Effectiveness and Efficiency* (Nuffield Provincial Hospitals Trust, London, 1972)

Coe, Rodney M. *Sociology of Medicine* (McGraw-Hill, London, 1970)

College of General Practitioners. 'Chronic Bronchitis in Great Britain', *British Medical Journal*, vol. 2 (1961), pp. 973-9

Collings, J.S. 'General Practice in England Today'. *Lancet*, i (1950), pp. 555-85

Department of Health and Social Security. *The Multiple Health Screening Clinic, Rotherham, 1966: A Social and Economic Assessment*, by J.L. Girt, L.A. Hooper and R.A. Abel, Reports on Public Health and Medical Subjects, no. 121 (HMSO, London, 1969)

Douglas, J.W.B. and Blomfield, J.M. *Children Under Five* (Allen and Unwin, London, 1958)

Dreitzel, Hans Peter. (ed.), *The Social Organization of Health* (Macmillan, New York, 1971)

Dunnell, Karen and Cartwright, Ann. *Medicine Takers, Prescribers and*

Hoarders (Routledge and Kegan Paul, London, 1972)

Eckstein, Harry. *The English Health Service: Its Origins, Structure and Achievements* (Harvard University Press, Cambridge, Mass., 1958)

Foote, Michael. *Aneurin Bevan: Volume Two, 1945-1960* (Davis-Poynter, London, 1973)

Forster, D.P. 'Social Class Differences in Sickness and General Practitioner Consultations', *Health Trends*, vol. 8, no. 2 (May 1976), pp. 29-32.

Forsyth, Gordon. *Doctors and State Medicine: A Study of the British Health Service* (Pitman Medical Publishing Co. Ltd, London, 1966)

Frankel, H. *Capitalist Society and Modern Sociology* (Lawrence and Wishart, London, 1970)

Friedson, Eliot. *Profession of Medicine: A Study of the Sociology of Applied Knowledge* (Harper and Row, New York, 1970)

Fry, J. *Medicine in Three Societies: A Comparison of Medical Care in the USSR, USA and UK* (American Elsevier Publishing Company, New York, 1970)

General Register Office. *The Registrar General's Decennial Supplement: England and Wales, 1961. Occupational Mortality* (HMSO, London, 1971)

———. *Regional and Social Factors in Infant Mortality*, by C.C. Spicer and L. Lipworth, Studies in Medical and Population Subjects, no. 19 (HMSO, London, 1966)

———. *Morbidity Statistics from General Practice*, by W.P.D. Logan and A.A. Cushion, Studies in Medical and Population Subjects, II, no. 14 (HMSO, London, 1960)

———. *The Registrar General's Decennial Supplement: England and Wales, 1951. Occupational Mortality*, part II, vol. 2 (HMSO, London, 1957)

———. *The Survey of Sickness, 1943-52*, by W.P.D. Logan and E.M. Brooke, Studies in Medical and Population Subjects, no. 12 (HMSO, London, 1957)

Gill, D.G. 'The British National Health Service: Professional Determinants of Administrative Structure', *International Journal of Health Services*, vol. 1, no. 4 (1971), pp. 342-53

Goldthorpe, John H. 'The Development of Social Policy in England, 1800-1914', *Transactions of the Fifth World Congress of Sociology*, vol. IV (1964)

Gosden, P.H.J.H. *The Friendly Societies in England* (Manchester University Press, Manchester, 1961)

Government Social Survey. *Diptheria Immunisation Inquiry*, by

P.G. Gray and A. Cartwright (HMSO, London, 1952)

——. *Survey of Sickness: October, 1943-December, 1945*, by
  P. Slater (HMSO, London, 1946)

Haberman, Paul W. 'The Reliability and Validity of the Data' in
  J. Kosa *et al. Poverty and Health* (Harvard University Press, Cambridge, Mass., 1969)

Halsey, A.H. (ed.), *Trends in British Society Since 1900: A Guide to the
  Changing Social Structure of Britain* (Macmillan, London, 1972)

Hart, Julian Tudor. 'Data on Occupational Mortality', *Lancet*, i (1972)

——, 'The Inverse Care Law', *Lancet*, i (1971), pp. 405-12

——, 'Health and Social Class', *Lancet*, i (1959), pp. 303-5

Herbert, S.M. *Britain's Health* (Penguin Books, Harmondsworth, 1939)

Hodgkinson, Ruth G. *The Origins of the National Health Service* (The
  Wellcome Historical Medical Library, London, 1967)

Holloway, S.W.F. 'Medical Education in England, 1830-1858: A Sociological Analysis', *History*, vol. 49 (October 1964)

Horn, J.S. *Away With All Pests* (Bantam, New York, 1972)

House of Commons, Expenditure Committee. *National Health Service
  Facilities for Private Patients* (HMSO, London, 1972)

Illich, Ivan. *Limits to Medicine* (McClelland and Stewart, Toronto,
  1976)

——. *Medical Nemesis* (McClelland and Stewart, Toronto, 1975)

Jay, D. *Socialism in the New Society* (Longmans, London, 1962)

Jewkes, J. and Jewkes, S. *Value for Money in Medicine* (Basil Blackwell,
  Oxford, 1963)

Johnson, Terence J. *Professions and Power* (Macmillan, London, 1972)

Kedward, H.B. 'Social Class Habits of Consulting', *British Journal of
  Preventive and Social Medicine*, vol. 16, no. 3 (1962), pp.147-52

Kessel, N. and Shepherd, M. 'The Health and Attitudes of People Who
  Seldom Consult a Doctor', *Medical Care*, vol. 3, no. 1 (1965),
  pp. 6-10

King Edward's Hospital Fund for London. *Provision for the Professional
  and Middle Classes at Voluntary Hospitals in London* (King Edward's
  Hospital Fund for London, London, 1936)

Krause, Elliott A. *Power and Illness: The Political Sociology of Health
  and Medical Care* (Elsevier, New York, 1977)

The Labour Party. *National Service for Health* (The Labour Party,
  London, 1943)

——. *The Hospital Problem* (The Labour Party, London, 1924)

——. Memoranda Prepared by the Advisory Committee on Public
  Health. I. *The Organisation of the Preventative and Curative Medical*

Services and Hospital and Laboratory Systems Under a Ministry of Health (The Labour Party, London, 1919)

Last, J.M. 'The Iceberg: Completing the Picture in General Practice', *Lancet*, ii (1963), pp. 28-31

Lee, M. *Opting out of the National Health Service* (Political and Economic Planning, London, 1971)

Lees, D.S. 'Private General Practice and the National Health Service', *Sociological Review*, Monograph no. 5 (July 1962), pp. 33-47

Leff, S. *The Health of the People* (Victor Gollancz, London, 1950)

Levy, H. *National Health Insurance* (Cambridge University Press, Cambridge, 1944)

Liang, Matthew H. *et al*. 'Chinese Health Care: Determinants of the System', *American Journal of Public Health*, vol. 63, no. 2 (February 1973), pp. 102-10

Lindsey, A. *Socialized Medicine in England and Wales* (University of North Carolina Press, Chapel Hill, NC, 1962)

Logan, W.P.D. 'Illness, Incapacity and Medical Attention Among Adults, 1947-49', *Lancet*, i (1950), pp. 773-6

Marsh, D.C. *The Changing Social Structure of England and Wales 1871-1961* Rev. edn (Routledge and Kegan Paul, London, 1965)

Mayer, T.C. 'Social Class and Health', *Update*, vol. 13, no. 10 (15 November 1976), pp. 1035, 1038-40

Mechanic, D. 'The English National Health Service: Some Comparisons with the United States', *Journal of Health and Social Behaviour*, vol. 12 (1971), pp. 18-29

Medical Planning Commission. 'Draft Interim Report', *British Medical Journal*, vol. 1 (1942), pp. 743-53

Medical Planning Research. 'Interim General Report', *Lancet*, ii (1942), pp. 599-622

Mencher, S. *Private Practice in Britain* (G. Bell and Sons, London, 1967)

Merrett, A.J. and Monk, D.A.G. 'The Structure of U.K. Taxation, 1962-63', *Bulletin of the Oxford University Institute of Economics and Statistics*, vol. 28, no. 3 (August 1966), pp. 145-62

McKeown, T. and C.R. Lowe. *An Introduction to Social Medicine*, 2nd edn (Blackwell, Oxford, 1974)

Miliband, R. *The State in Capitalist Society* (Quartet, London, 1969)

Miller, F.J.W. *et al. Growing up in Newcastle-upon-Tyne* (Oxford University Press, London, 1960)

Ministry of Health. Consultative Council on Medical and Allied Services. *Interim Report on the Future Provision of Medical and Allied*

Services Cmd. 693 (HMSO, London, 1920)

—— and General Register Office. *Reports of Hospital Inpatient Enquiry for the Two Years 1960 and 1961*, part III (HMSO, London, 1967)

Morris, J.N. 'Priorities in the Health Service' in P. Draper, M. Kogan and J.N. Morris, *The NHS: Three Views*, Fabian Society Research Series, no. 287 (Fabian Society, London, 1970)

Morris, J.N. and Heady, J.A. 'Social and Biological Factors in Infant Mortality: V. Mortality in Relation to Father's Occupation, 1911-1950', *Lancet*, i (1955), pp. 554-9

——. 'The National Health Service Act in Great Britain.' *The Practitioner*, vol. 163 (1949)

Navarro, Vicente. *Class Struggle, The State and Medicine* (Martin Robertson, London, 1978)

——. 'Social Class, Political Power and the State and Their Implications in Medicine', *Social Science and Medicine*, vol. 10 (1976), pp. 437-57

——. 'The Industrialization of Fetishism or the Fetishism of Industrialization: A Critique of Ivan Illich', *Social Science and Medicine*, vol. 9 (1975), pp. 351-63

Nicholson, J.L. 'Redistribution of Income in the United Kingdom in 1959, 1957 and 1953' in C. Clark and G. Stuvel (eds.), *Income and Wealth*, Series X (Bowes and Bowes, London, 1964)

Nuffield Provincial Hospitals Trust. *The Hospital Surveys: The Domesday Book of the Hospital Services* (University Press, Oxford, 1946)

Office of Population Censuses and Surveys. *The General Household Survey, 1975* (HMSO, London, 1978)

——. *Occupational Mortality. The Registrar General's Decennial Supplement for England and Wales, 1970-72* (HMSO, London, 1978)

——. *The General Household Survey, 1974* (HMSO, London, 1977)

——. *The General Household Survey* (HMSO, London, 1973)

Oppenheim, A. 'Dental Charges: A Survey of the Means Test at Work', *Cambridge Poverty*, no. 3 (January 1972), pp. 4-5

Osborn, G.R. and Leyshon, V.N. 'Domiciliary Testing of Cervical Smears by Home Nurses', *Lancet*, i (1966), pp. 256-7

Parker, Julia. *Social Policy and Citizenship* (Macmillan, London, 1975)

Pinker, Robert, *English Hospital Statistics 1861-1938* (Heinemann, London, 1966)

Pivan, Frances Fox and Richard A. Cloward. *Regulating the Poor: The Functions of Public Welfare* (Pantheon Books, New York, 1971)

Political and Economic Planning. *Family Needs and The Social Services*

(Allen and Unwin, London, 1961)

Rein, M. 'Social Class and the Utilization of Medical Care Services', *Hospitals*, vol. 43 (1 July 1969), pp. 43-54

Renaud, Marc. 'On the Structural Constraints to State Intervention in Health', *International Journal of Health Services*, vol. 5, no. 4 (1975), pp. 559-71

Review Body of Doctors' and Dentists' Remuneration. *Fourth Report*, 1974, Cmd. 5644 (HMSO, London, 1974)

Rifkin, S.B. 'Public Health in China — Is the Experience Relevant to Other Less Developed Nations?', *Social Science and Medicine*, vol. 7 (1973), pp. 249-57

Rose, A. *The Power Structure* (Oxford University Press, New York, 1967)

Ross, D. Reid. 'National Health Service in Factorytown: A Survey of the Demand for Medical Care in an Industrial Community', *Medical World*, vol. 78, no. 2 (1953), pp. 125-38

Rossdale, M. 'Socialist Health Service?', *New Left Review*, no. 36 (1966), pp. 3-25

——. 'Health in a Sick Society', *New Left Review*, no. 34 (1965), pp. 82-91

Royal Commission on National Health Insurance. *Report* (HMSO, London, 1926)

Royal Commission on the Poor Laws and Relief of Distress. *Report*, vol. 1 (HMSO, London, 1909)

Runciman, W.G. *Relative Deprivation and Social Justice* (Routledge and Kegan Paul, London, 1966)

Sidel, V.W. 'Some Observations on the Health Services in the People's Republic of China', *International Journal of Health Services*, vol. 2, no. 3 (1972), pp. 385-95

Socialist Medical Association. *The Socialist Programme for Health* (Socialist Medical Association, London, 1943)

——. *A Socialised Medical Service* (Socialist Medical Association, London, 1933)

Spence, J. *et al. A Thousand Families in Newcastle-upon-Tyne* (Oxford University Press, London, 1954)

Stark Murray, D. *Why a National Health Service?* (Pemberton Books, London, 1971)

Stein, L. 'Morbidity in a London General Practice: Social and Demographic Data.' *British Journal of Preventive and Social Medicine*, vol. 14, no. 1 (1960), pp. 9-15

Strachey, J. *Contemporary Capitalism* (Victor Gollancz, London, 1956)

Susser, M.W. and Watson, W. *Sociology in Medicine*, 2nd edn (Oxford University Press, London, 1971)

Swartz, Donald. 'The Politics of Reform: Conflict and Accommodation in Canadian Health Policy' in Leo Panitch (ed.), *The Canadian State* (University of Toronto Press, Toronto, 1977)

Taylor, S.J.L. *Good General Practice* (Oxford University Press, London, 1954)

Titmuss, Richard M. *Problems of Social Policy* (HMSO, London, 1976)

——. *The Gift Relationship* (Allen and Unwin, London, 1970)

——. 'Role of the Family Doctor Today in the Context of Britain's Social Services', *Lancet*, i (1965), pp. 1-4

——. *Essays on the Welfare State* (Unwin University Books, London, 1963)

——. 'Health' in Morris Ginsberg (ed.), *Law and Opinion in England in the 20th Century* (University of California Press, Berkeley, 1959)

The Trades Union Congress and the Labour Party. *The Labour Movement and Preventive and Curative Medical Services: A Statement of Policy With Regard to Health* (The Trades Union Congress and the Labour Party, London, 1923)

——. *The Labour Movement and the Hospital Crisis: A Statement of Policy With Regard to Hospitals* (The Trades Union Congress and the Labour Party, London, 1922)

Tuckett, D. *An Introduction to Medical Sociology* (Tavistock, London, 1976)

U.K. Private Medical Care: Provident Schemes Statistics, 1977 (Lee Donaldson Associates, London, 1978)

U.K. Private Medical Care: Provident Schemes Statistics, 1976 (Lee Donaldson Associates, London, 1977)

US Department of Health, Education and Welfare, Public Health Service, National Centre for Health Statistics. *Conceptual Problems in Developing an Index of Health*, Vital and Health Statistics, series 2, no. 17 (Government Printing Office, Washington, DC, 1966)

Watkins, Brian. *Documents on Health and Social Services: 1834 to the Present Day* (Methuen, London, 1975)

Webb, B. and Webb, S. *The State and the Doctor* (Longmans, Green and Co., London, 1910)

Webb, S. and Webb, B. (eds.), *The Break-up of the Poor Law* (Longmans, Green and Co., London, 1909)

Wedderburn, Dorothy. (ed.), *Poverty Inequality and Class Structure* (Cambridge University Press, London, 1974)

——. 'Facts and Theories of the Welfare State', *The Socialist Register*

(1965), pp. 127-46

Weinstein, J. *The Corporate Ideal in the Liberal State* (Beacon Press, Boston, 1968)

Westergaard, John and Resler, Henrietta. *Class in a Capitalist Society* (Penguin, Harmondsworth, 1976)

Wilensky, H.L. *The Welfare State and Equality* (University of California Press, Berkeley, 1975)

Willcocks, Arthur J. *The Creation of the National Health Service* (Routledge and Kegan Paul, London, 1967)

——. ' "A Process of Erosion?": Pressure Groups and the National Health Service Act of 1946', *Sociological Review*, Monograph no. 5 (July 1962), pp. 9-19

INDEX

Abel-Smith, Brian 44n1, n3, n16,
45nn22-3, n25, n29, n30, nn33-5,
n37, 46n59, n63, 58, 59nn2-4,
60nn11-15, n18, n33, n36, n47,
96, 103n72, 113n13, 142, 143,
155n20
access to care, under the National
Health Service *see* quality of care,
use of National Health Service
Acheson, Roy M. 141n28
Aird, Lesley 141n28
Airth, A.D. 145, 154n5
Alderson, M.R. 145, 154n7, n8
Andersen, R. 154n11
Anderson, Sir John 104
Annas, George J. 73n5
Ashford, J.R. 131, 140n8, 142,
154n2
Ashley, J.S.A. 148, 155n15, n16
autonomy, of medical profession
76-8, 95, 97

Bacon, Robert 73n3
Bain, George Sayer 73n2
Barr, A. 143, 145, 154n4
Bendix, R. 45n19
Bevan, Aneurin 85, 99, 105, 113n8
Beveridge, Sir William 66, 70, 75n44
Birmingham and Midland Ear and
Throat Hospital 53
Birmingham Contributory Scheme 51
Birnbaum, N. 22n2
Blomfield, J.M. 128n29
Bonham, D.G. 146, 154n8
Brand, Jeanne L. 79, 101n7, n12
British Hospitals Association 58, 83
British Institute of Public Opinion
104, 113n3
British Medical Association: attitudes
towards hospital contributory
schemes 34; attitudes towards
pay beds 37, 52; co-operation
with Trades Union Congress 67-8;
opposition to National Health
Service 99; proposals for reform
85-6

British Provident Association 37
British United Provident Association
149, 150
Brown, Ernest 98
Bruce, M. 44n1, n7
Butler, N.R. 146, 154n8

Cartwright, Ann 126, 128n23, n28,
130, 134, 136-9, 140n3, n4,
141n12, nn16-21, n28, 148,
154n14, 155n17, n18
Cave Committee 50, 51, 57
class conflict, and social welfare
legislation 16-19, 47, 61-2
class relations *see* social class
Cloward, Richard A. 19, 23nn11-13,
59n1
Cochrane, A.L. 21, 23n21
Coe, Rodney M. 25, 44n4, 101n1
College of General Practitioners 126,
128n27, 138
Collings, J.S. 138, 139, 141n23, n27
Consultative Council on Medical and
Allied Services 79, 81, 88-9, 99,
101n14, 102n29, n50, n51,
103n55

Dawson Report *see* Consultative
Council on Medical and Allied
Services
destitute, care available for 26-8
Douglas, J.W.B. 128n29
Dreitzel, Hans Peter 74n5, 103n78,
161n8
Dunnell, Karen 126, 128n28, 131,
140n4

Eckstein, Harry 60n8, n10, n35, n38,
88, 98, 102n53, 103n70, nn80-2
Eichling, Philip S. 73n5
Emergency Hospital Service 83
Emergency Medical Service 54, 99
Eyer, Joseph 161n7

family clubs 42
Fine, Lawrence J. 73n5

Foote, Michael 85, 102n44, n45
Forster, D.P. 140n10
Forsyth, Gordon 88, 96, 101n7,
    102n52, 103n73, n75, n76, n80,
    116, 127n5, 154n12, n13
Frankel, H. 20, 23n16
Freeman, H.E. 161n5
Friedson, Eliot 46n64, 77, 101nn4-6,
    103n78, n83, 162n8
friendly societies 26, 42

General Household Survey 124, 125,
    128n24, n25, 132, 133-4, 136,
    140nn9-11
general practitioner care: class differ-
    ences in consultations 108-12,
    129-37; class differences in
    quality of 137-9
general practitioners: income 96-7;
    isolation and low status 83-4;
    uneven distribution 56-7, 113n9
Ginsberg, Morris 101n8
Goldsthorpe, John H. 22n1
Gosden, P.H.J.H. 44n5, n6
Graham, Saxon 161n5
Guy's Hospital 35, 36, 48

Haberman, Paul W. 127n3
Halsey, A.H. 73n3
Hart, Julian Tudor 21, 23n27,
    113n9, 140n2
Hastings, Dr Somerville 71, 94
Herbert, S.M. 40, 42, 45n29, n36,
    46n67, n69
Hodgkinson, Ruth G. 27, 44n1, 78,
    101nn9-11
Holloway, S.W.F. 44n2, 45n18, n20,
    n21
Horn, J.S. 73n5
Hospital Inpatient Enquiry 142-3,
    154n1
Hospital Savings Association 34, 37,
    51
hospitals, pre-National Health
    Service: class composition 31-2;
    growth of contributory schemes
    33-4, 50-2; increasing costs of
    providing care 47-9; introduction
    of charges 32-3; lack of co-
    ordination 55, 57-8; provision of
    pay beds 35-8; quality of care
    25-6, 31, 35; size 49; uneven
    distribution of services 55-6, *see
    also* Poor Law, voluntary

hospitals
House, James S. 161n7

ideas, as source of change 16
Illich, Ivan 45n17, 103n78, 127n2,
    161n5
illness: as an individual responsibility
    158-9; changing attitudes
    towards 30; social and political
    bases 159-60, *see also* morbidity
    rates, mortality rates
income redistribution 24-5
individualism, and increasing concern
    with health 30

Jay, D. 20, 22n3, 23n15, 161n3
Jewkes, J. and S. 128n22
Johnson, Terence J. 96, 103n74, 79

Kedward, H.B. 131, 140n5
Kessel, N. 131, 140n6
King Edward's Hospital Fund for
    London: annual statistical
    review for 1931 52; attitudes to
    pay beds 36, 37; contributions to
    53; co-ordination of voluntary
    hospitals 57; grants to voluntary
    hospitals 50
Kohn, Robert 161n4
Kosa, J. 127n3
Krause, Elliott 101n1, 161n7

Labour Party: Advisory Committee
    on Public Health 79, 80, 82, 90;
    evolution of policy on health
    services 70-2
Lalonde, Marc 161n5
Last, J.M. 116, 127n4
Lee, M. 155n22, n24
Lees, D.S. 155n19
Leff, S. 44n12, 60n42
Levine, S. 161n5
Levy, H. 46n65, n70
Leyshon, V.N. 141n14
Liang, Matthew H. 73n5
Lindsey, A. 45n32, 60n6, 41,
    113n12
Liverpool Workpeople's Hospital Fund
    51
Lloyd George 39, 78, 79
Local Government Act 45n29
Logan, W.P.D. 128n21
London Fever Hospital 50
London Hospital 32, 36, 48, 54

Lowe, C.R. 44n15, 161n7

McKeown, T. 44n15, 161n7
Manchester Royal Infirmary 36, 50
Mechanic, D. 21, 23n23, 108, 113n15, 140n2
medical clubs 26
Medical Planning Commission 79, 83-4, 86-8, 93, 97, 102n18, n35, n39, n49, 103n67, n77, 112n1
Medical Planning Research 80, 81, 83, 91-2, 102n19, n26, n27, n37, n39, 103n64
medical profession: attitudes towards pay beds 50-2; criticisms of health services 80-4; definitions of illness and role of medicine 84; early support for state medical services 78-9; opposition to National Health Service 98-100; proposals for a national health service 85-92, areas of dispute 85, reactions 93-4; state medical services and interests of 76-9, 95-8
medicine: effect on health 15, 28-9, 39, 44n15, n17; increasing sophistication 30; political bases 97-8, 159-60
Mencher, S. 150, 153, 155n26, n29, n35, n37
Metropolitan Asylums Board 32
Metropolitan Poor Act 31, 32
middle class patients, before 1948: increasing costs of care 37; problems in obtaining hospital care 35-9; quality of care 28-9; sources of care in mid-nineteenth century 24-5, *see also* quality of care, use of National Health Service
Miliband, R. 18, 20, 22n2, n6, 23n17, 59n1, 73n1
Miller, F.J.W. 128n29
morbidity rates: class differences in 123-6; limitations as a measure of needs for care 116-17
mortality rates: class differences in 117-23; limitations as a measure of needs for care 115-16

National Health Insurance; attitudes of Trades Union Congress 62-6; limitations 39-42
National Health Service: assumed
reduction of class inequality 20-1; explanations of introduction of 18-19; lack of critical research 21, 129, 139-40, 148, 154; rationalisation of health services 47, 100, 104-6, 157
National Hospital 50
Navarro, Vicente 18, 19, 20, 22n2, n8, n9, 23n10, n18, 59n1, 61, 73n1, n2, 76, 101n2, 103n83
needs for care, problems in identifying 115, *see also* morbidity rates, mortality rates
Newell, D.J. 145, 154n5
Nightingale, Florence 25
Nottingham General Hospital 36
Nuffield Provincial Hospitals Trust 45n51, 60n39, n43, n48
nursing homes 38

Osborn, G.R. 141n14
O'Toole, James 161n7

Parker, Julia 21, 23n25, n26
Pearson, M.G. 131, 140n8, 142, 154n2
physician's fees, graded in relation to income 24-5
Pimlott, John 73n3
Pinker, Robert 51, 60n5, n7, n22
Pivan, Francis Fox 19, 23n11, n12, n13, 59n1
Player, J.D. 36
pluralist theories 17, 158-9
Political and Economic Planning 34, 125, 128n26, 142, 154n3
Poor Law Amendment Act 31
Poor Law, care available under 25-8, 31-4
private medical care schemes 149-51; impact on National Health Service care 151-3
Private Patients Plan 149
provident dispensaries 26
provident medical associations 26, 42

quality of care, class differences in: general practitioner 137-9; hospital 147-9, 151-3

Reeder, L.G. 161n5
Rein, M. 21, 23n22, 140n2
Renaud, Marc 74n5, 103n79, 161n5
Resler, Henrietta 23n28, 161n6

Rifkin, S.B. 73n5
Rose, A. 22n3
Ross, D. Reid 113n17
Rossdale, M. 21, 23n24, 74n5,
    103n78, 162n8
Royal College of Physicians 24, 86
Royal College of Surgeons 24, 29, 86
Royal Commission on National
    Health Insurance 43, 46n68, 99
Royal Commission on the Poor Laws
    33, 45n26, n27, n28
Royal Northern Hospital 53
Runciman, W.G. 73n3

St Bartholomew's Hospital 48
St Mary's Hospital 35
St Thomas's Hospital 35
Sheffield Royal Infirmary 48
Shepherd, M. 131, 140n6
Sidel, V.W. 73n5
Smiles, Samuel 30
Social class: and illness 159-60;
    definition 23n28; morbidity rates
    123-6; mortality rates 117-23;
    Registrar General's classification
    127n7, *see also* middle class,
    quality of care, upper class,
    use of National Health Service,
    working class
Socialist Medical Association:
    proposals for reform 90-1; role in
    development of Labour Party
    policy 71, 72
social welfare legislation: assumed
    effect on class inequality 20-1;
    explanations of growth of 16-19,
    61
Spence, J. 128n29
state: arguments in House of
    Commons for National Health
    Service 105-6; as mediator 17, 18;
    ideological function 15, 160;
    legitimation of class inequality
    160; response to delegations from
    Trades Union Congress 64, 65, 69
Stein, L. 131, 140n7
Sterling, Peter 161n7
Strachey, J. 17, 21, 22n4, n5, 23n19,
    59n1, 73n1, 161n3
Survey of Sickness 109-12, 113n18,
    n19, n22, 124-5, 128n18, n19,
    n20, 131-3, 136
Susser, M.W. 101n1, n4, 128n16
Swansea Hospital 52

Taylor, S.J.L. 138, 139, 141n22, n24,
    n25, n29
Titmuss, Richard M. 21, 23n20, 53,
    60n9, n31, n37, n40, n49, n50,
    78, 101n8, 113n13, 139, 141n26,
    142, 143, 146, 154n9, n10
Trades Union Congress: co-operation
    with British Medical Association
    67-8; criticisms of health services
    62-6; lack of co-operation with
    Socialist Medical Association 67-8;
    late consideration of comprehen-
    sive reform of health services
    66-70

upper class, sources of care in mid-
    nineteenth century 24-5
use of National Health Service, class
    differences in: general practitioners
    129-37; hospitals 142-6; immed-
    iate impact of National Health
    Service 108-12; preventive care
    134, 136; problems in interpreting
    data 136-7, 147

voluntary hospitals 25, 27; class
    composition 32; expenditures 49;
    financial crises 49-50, 52-4;
    introduction of charges 32-3;
    sources of revenue 33, 51-2
Voluntary Hospitals Commission 58

Watkins, Brian 102n54
Watson, W. 101n1, n4, 128n16
Webb, Sidney and Beatrice 27, 28,
    44n1, n9, n11, n13, n14, 45n24
Wedderburn, Dorothy 18, 22n7,
    59n1, 73n1
Weinstein, J. 22n2, 23n14
welfare state *see* social welfare legis-
    lation
Westergaard, John 23n28, 161n6
Westminster Hospital 33
White, Kerr L. 161n4
Willcocks, Arthur J. 103n80
Willink, Henry 99, 105
working class patients, before 1948:
    increasing demand for hospital
    care 31-2; quality of care 28-9;
    sources of care in mid-nineteenth
    century 25-8, *see also* quality of
    care, use of National Health
    Service